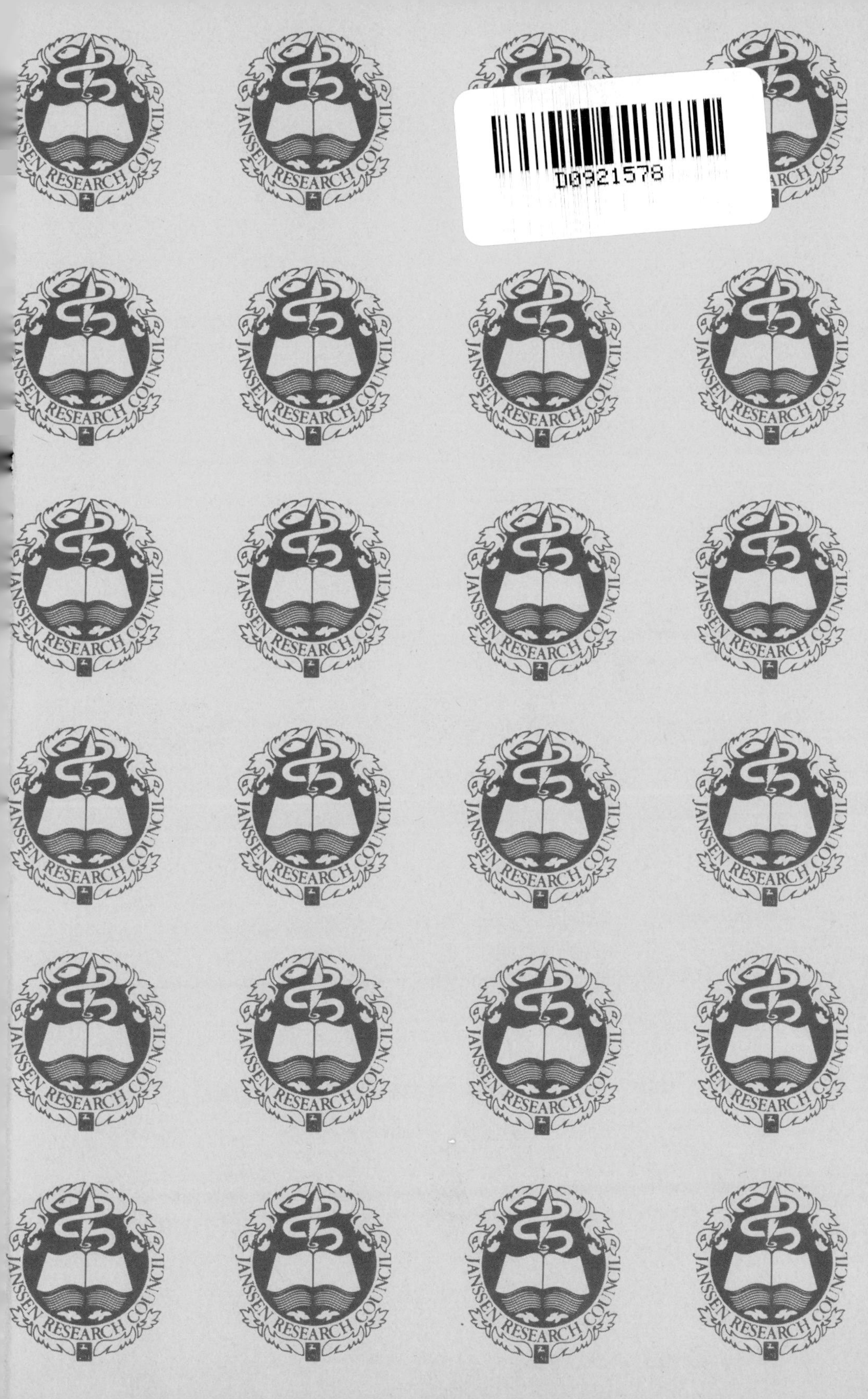
JANSSEN RESEARCH COUNCIL
D0921578

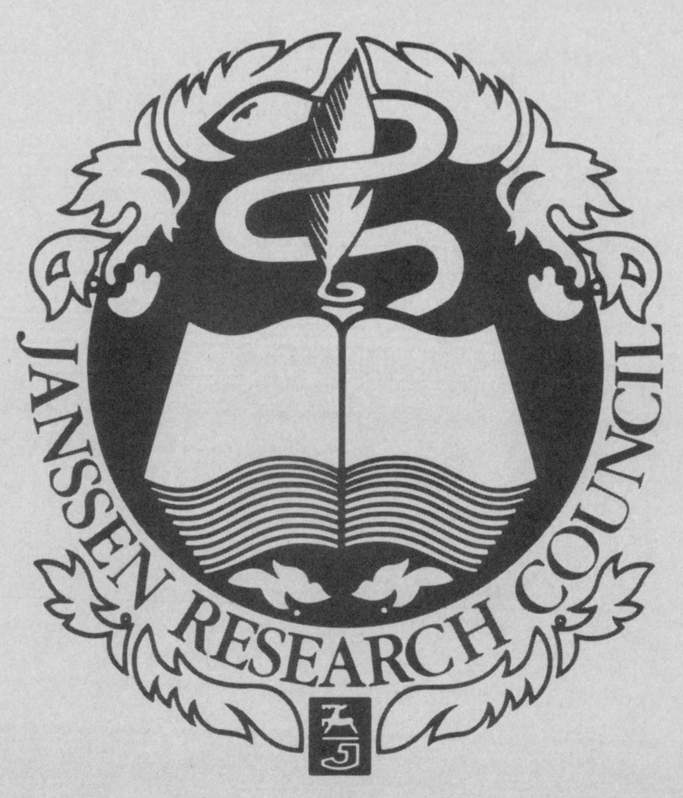
JANSSEN RESEARCH COUNCIL

Breakthrough

The Discovery of Modern Medicines at Janssen

Breakthrough

The Discovery of Modern Medicines at Janssen

Harry Schwartz

Afterword by Jack B. McConnell, M.D.

The Skyline Publishing Group
New Jersey

Edited by William J. McGuire

Printing History 9 8 7 6 5 4 3 2

Library of Congress Cataloging-in-Publication Data

Schwartz, Harry, 1919-
Breakthrough: the discovery of modern medicines at Janssen/ Harry Schwartz.
p. cm.
ISBN 1-56019-100-7: $24.95
1. Janssen, Paul A. J. (Paul Adreiaan Jan), 1926-
2. Pharmacologists--Belgium--Biography. 3. Chemistry. Pharmaceutical--Research. 4. Janssen Pharmaceutica--History.
I. Title.
RS73.J33S38 1990
615'.1'092--dc20 90-61712
[B] CIP

Printed in U.S.A.

The following trademarks of Johnson & Johnson and its affiliated companies appear in this book:

ALFENTA, CLINACOX, DIPIPERON, FENTANYL, HALDOL, HISMANAL, IMODIUM, IMPROMEN, INAPSINE, INNOVAR, MICATIN, MONISTAT, NIZORAL, ORAP, PALFIUM, PREPULSID, REASEC, REMIVOX, SIBELIUM, SPARTRIX, STUGERON, SUBLIMAZE, SUFENTA, TILT, TINSET, VERMOX.

To My Grandchildren
Aaron, Daniel, Mark, David, Bonnie and Stephanie

PHOTO CREDITS

The Image Bank:
- Morton Beebe
- Derek Berwin
- Kay Chernush
- Lawrence Fried
- Guido Rossi
- Jules Zalon

Janssen Pharmaceutica

Johnson & Johnson

The Record:
- Ed Hill

William Strode Associates:
- William Strode

ACKNOWLEDGMENTS

I wish to express my appreciation to those who have helped me write this book. In particular, I would like to thank Dr. Paul Janssen, who repeatedly made himself available and patiently answered my numerous questions.

To Dr. Janssen's associates, especially Robert Stouthuysen, Lucien Wauters, Dr. Robert Marsboom, Dr. Marcel Janssen, Dr. Marcel Borgers, Viviane Schuermans, Karel Schellekens, Dr. Jan Van Cutsem, Dr. Cyriel Van der Eycken, Dr. Jan Heeres, Dr. Josee Leysen, Dr. Willem Van Bever, Dr. Jozef Heykants, Dr. Carlos Niemegeers, Dr. Albert Wauquier, Dr. Frans Awouters, Dr. Anton Jageneau, Dr. Hugo Vanden Bossche, Dr. Oscar Vanparijs, Dr. Andre Reyntjens, Dr. Gabriel Vanden Bussche, Dr. Staf Van Gestel, Dr. Hubert Hermans, Ludovicus Smit, Francois Van De Craen, Andre Janssens, Alex Op De Beeck.

To Dr. Ajit Shetty, past president of Janssen Pharmaceutica USA; Dr. David Shand, senior vice president of United States research for the Janssen Research Foundation; and Dr. Richard Wildnauer, for their cooperation.

To Lawrence G. Foster, corporate vice president of public relations of Johnson & Johnson, who facilitated this unprecedented effort to tell the research story of a major creative pharmaceutical firm.

To Roger Aspeling, director of professional relations of Janssen Pharmaceutica USA, who has been my constant and indispensable guide during my fascinating journey through the creative world of Janssen.

Finally, I am in great debt to my wife, Ruth, who prepared the index for this book, and who for three years has cheerfully and competently acted as wife, research assistant and domestic psychiatrist as I wrestled to learn what the men and women of Janssen have done, and to translate that knowledge into words that would appeal to the curious public.

Harry Schwartz
November 1989

AUTHOR'S NOTE

This book had its birth in my ignorance and my curiosity. For many years I have had to become more familiar with medical matters — my own and my family's — than I would have liked. Throughout these experiences, I wondered where medicines came from.

I, my wife, and our children have repeatedly benefited from using a long list of pharmaceuticals as our needs dictated. But it was exasperating to learn that my doctors knew no more about the making of medicines than I did. Of course they and I knew the origins of a few medicines, notably insulin (Banting and Best), penicillin (Alexander Fleming) and streptomycin (Selman Waksman). But these drugs were atypical. The origins of almost all other drugs are as unknown as the identity of the farmer whose cow provides the milk we drink.

After a long and varied career, I became a writer on pharmaceutical topics, or, to be more explicit, a columnist for the United States magazine *Pharmaceutical Executive* and the international pharmaceutical newsletter *Scrip*. I took advantage of this opportunity to ask the pharmaceutical industry why it seemed to keep secret the origins of the medicines which were its stock in trade. I suggested repeatedly that if intelligent and concerned citizens knew more about the enormous effort, time, and money that go into producing new and better medicines, there might be more public appreciation for the pharmaceutical industry's contributions and its problems.

On one occasion, I wrote about the lack of publicly known heroes of the pharmaceutical industry. In a prominent place on my list was the Belgian researcher Dr. Paul A. Janssen.

Dr. Janssen, whom I had not met at that time, excited my interest because he and his collaborators at Janssen Pharmaceutica had, since 1953, discovered and made available more new medicines than any other similar group of researchers in the world. I asked the obvious questions: What was there about the Janssen research approach that produced these dazzling results? Could other pharmaceutical companies learn something from Dr. Janssen and his colleagues and make better progress if they emulated them?

It was this writing that brought me into personal contact with Dr. Janssen. He invited me to lunch in Washington, D.C., during one of his visits to the United States. I accepted the invitation with alacrity and had the opportunity to ask my questions and get his answers.

Simply put, Dr. Janssen believed that if there was any secret to his firm's greater productivity, it lay primarily in the lack of bureaucracy at Janssen Pharmaceutica. He said his door was always open to his researchers who might want to consult him. His firm did not have a top-heavy apparatus of committees that often wasted so much time and energy, and slowed up the real work.

In my meeting with Dr. Janssen, I reiterated my interest in helping people learn more about how drugs are actually discovered. Dr. Janssen thought that notion made sense. Out of that discussion came the idea for this book, which is an attempt to present accurately, and as simply as possible, the story of how Janssen Pharmaceutica made a number of its most important discoveries which are now helping people all over the world.

I have attempted to sketch the logic of Janssen research and development. The chemical diagrams or structural formulas which pepper the pages of this book are simply an aid to comprehension. I have described the compounds as they appear in the two-dimensional diagrams. The complex chemistry involved in the Janssen achievements has been omitted since it cannot be readily communicated to the intelligent but nontechnical reader.

Harry Schwartz
Scarsdale, N.Y.
November 15, 1989

TABLE OF CONTENTS

FOREWORD

For those who are fascinated by watching important things happen, living in the last two-thirds of the twentieth century has truly been a stroke of good fortune. For the relatively few with the talent and the opportunity to make important things happen, the same period of time has been richly rewarding -- both for themselves and for humanity. Paul Janssen is one of those contributors.

No area of human endeavor has seen more dramatic improvement during this century than has medical and pharmaceutical research. Not too many years ago the physician's entire armamentarium of medicines was carried in his leather valise. He struggled to make sick people well, often against hopeless odds. Then came the dawn of the age of miracle drugs and a burst of new discoveries from pharmaceutical research laboratories.

Being responsible for one or more important new pharmaceutical compounds, in itself, is a significant accomplishment. But researching and developing seventy new pharmaceuticals over a span of thirty-six years is a remarkable achievement without precedent in the pharmaceutical industry. That distinction belongs to Paul Janssen and his research team at Beerse, Belgium. Five of these compounds are on the "essential drug" list compiled by the World Health Organization in Geneva, Switzerland.

No pharmaceutical scientist since the invention of antibiotics has had a broader impact on world health than has Dr. Janssen. He has developed pioneering compounds in the fields of mycology, parasitology, psychiatry, gastroenterology, and blood circulation, and in doing so, solved some of the world's most perplexing health problems.

It all had a storybook beginning. Back in 1961 Johnson & Johnson, which itself had pioneered the science of sterility in wound care, courted and won the respect of the young and promising Janssen Pharmaceutica. It turned out to be an incredibly farsighted decision for both companies. Johnson & Johnson had set its sights on becoming a major factor in pharmaceuticals, and Janssen needed resources and the clout of a major marketing organization in the health care field. Over time, both organizations realized their objectives, and certainly untold numbers of patients have benefited.

Paul Janssen once defined research as "the things one does to satisfy one's curiosity." That suggests some of the intrigue in store for the readers in these pages. Just as the bringing together of the Janssen and Johnson & Johnson organizations was a fortuitous event, so was the decision to have author Harry Schwartz write this book. Few authors are as well qualified to take such an intrinsically complex subject as pharmaceutical research and turn it into readable, accurate, and appealing prose as he has done. The journalist in Dr. Schwartz comes to the forefront in *Breakthrough*, and the reader is rewarded with a highly informative and enjoyable experience.

*Lawrence G. Foster
New Brunswick, New Jersey
October 15, 1989

*Mr. Foster is corporate vice president
of public relations for Johnson & Johnson
and author of *A Company That Cares*,
the 100-year history of Johnson & Johnson

Chapter 1

MOLECULES TO MEDICINE

Physicians like to point out, and rightly, how much better and more powerful modern medicine is than the medicine practiced in the eras of our fathers and grandfathers. The physicians of those earlier years were undoubtedly just as intelligent and just as interested in helping their patients as today's physicians. But doctors now know far more about the human body than their predecessors did and, no less important, have a far larger armory of weapons to use against disease.

Most of those weapons are medicines of the most diverse kinds; medicines that have been discovered since the end of World War II. It is these medicines that are largely responsible for the vast improvements in world health since the middle of this century, the great increase in the average life span, the sharp fall in infant mortality, and the major improvements in the quality of life enjoyed by hundreds of millions of people.

Just in the past thirty years or so, we have eliminated smallpox, historically one of the world's great killers. Polio, once a mass killer and crippler of the young, has now become so rare that most younger doctors in developed countries have never seen a victim of this disease. Kidney failure was, not so long ago, a guarantee of quick death. Today, kidney dialysis and kidney transplants permit hundreds of thousands of people to live quite satisfactory lives even after their own kidneys have ceased functioning. The traditional infectious diseases — tuberculosis, cholera, pneumonia, scarlet fever — were once mass killers of young and old. Now, they are rare among most population groups because antibiotics and other medicines can, in most cases, cure them.

Syphilis and gonorrhea, once the scourge of millions, are now cured so easily that they are no longer regarded as major health problems. The conquest of these sexually transmitted diseases, plus the ability of oral contraceptives to separate procreation from recreation, contributed to a sexual revolution of enormous dimensions.

Modern medicine has also provided the drugs now available against acute and chronic pain; medicines that have revolutionized psychiatry and eased emotional distress; more effective weapons against fungal and viral diseases; new anesthetics that have widened the arena in which the surgeon's knife is useful. In addition, come the promises of biotechnology, whose first products have already revolutionized diagnosis, and whose first therapeutic drugs are saving the lives of some people and improving the quality of life for many others.

All of these advances have occurred in a relatively short period of time. In 1910, when Paul Ehrlich discovered his "magic bullet" against syphilis, the world hailed his achievement. Shortly after World War I, two Canadians, Frederick Banting and Charles Best, became household names when their discovery of insulin showed how the lives of diabetics could be extended by many years. Two decades later, the discovery of penicillin, the first antibiotic, brought world-wide fame and the Nobel Prize to Alexander Fleming, Ernst Chain, and Howard Florey.

Against this background, the modern research pharmaceutical industry quickly developed in the industrialized countries after World War II. It began to discover and produce many effective new medicines. Occasionally, the public has caught a glimpse of the personal drama behind drug discoveries among rival individuals or teams, as when Jonas Salk and Albert Sabin contested the issue of whose polio vaccine was better, or when Robert Gallo and Luc Montagnier debated over which one of them had discovered the virus that causes acquired immune deficiency syndrome (AIDS).

Yet, as in so many other fields, the success of drugs and the medical profession has brought indifference and even complaints. We have reenacted the roller coaster ride in public response observed in the field of space. The first sputniks filled us with awe; the pictures of the first men walking on the moon made us realize what an age of marvels we lived in. But too soon yesterday's miracles became today's routine. Space achievement after space achievement brought only yawns.

Then suddenly and unexpectedly, catastrophe wrenched our bored perspectives into a more realistic context. The Challenger explosion brutally reminded us how remarkable it has been that all the earlier space shuttle flights had gone so well despite the terrible dangers which were always a possibility. What the Challenger disaster did for space research, the tragedy of AIDS, killing thousands of young people in the prime of their lives, has done for medicine. All of a sudden we hear a clamor. Where are the new drugs needed to save the lives of AIDS patients and to prevent the further spread of the disease?

A public accustomed to the idea that we had or would soon have all the drugs needed to combat disease looked on in amazement as it became clear that we had no effective remedies against AIDS. No one could predict with any real confidence when we might have them. For the first time, it occurred to millions that essential drugs do not fall free from heaven, like the Biblical manna, but have to be searched for, discovered, and developed at enormous effort and very great cost.

When the drug Retrovir (AZT) showed it could prolong the lives of AIDS victims, it was first hailed with gratitude. But then, as it became known how expensive the AZT treatment would be, there was grumbling. Voices began asking why this drug had to cost so much. Legislators who, before AZT's discovery, had proposed spending billions of dollars annually on research for anti-AIDS drugs, suddenly began complaining. Angrily, they pointed out that it would cost millions of dollars each year to treat AIDS victims with this expensive drug, which lengthened a patient's life but did not cure this terminal disease.

The AIDS tragedy has pointed out several things: first, that new diseases can appear without warning at any time; second, that the increased power of medicines has sometimes brought with it unrealistic expectations; and, third, that the discovery and synthesis of new drugs is never an overnight achievement.

But exactly how are new medicines discovered and made available to patients? There is obviously no one simple and direct route. Every new pharmaceutical has its own particular complex biography. But in general, effective new medicines are what the chemists call organic compounds. They consist of molecules which have carbon as well as other atoms. Carbon compounds are the chemistry of life. At the most elementary level, we breathe in oxygen and breathe out carbon dioxide. Plants take in carbon dioxide and give off oxygen. But carbon dioxide is one of the simplest organic compounds. Most of the carbon compounds that make possible the normal operation of the human organism are far more complicated.

No one can study the chemistry of life without developing a sense of awe at its enormous complexity and flawless functioning under normal conditions. Every second, a huge number of carbon compounds in our bodies are formed and broken down, then formed and broken down again, in the ceaseless cycle of chemical reactions called life.

All living creatures are effectively autonomous chemical factories producing carbon compounds needed for growth, repair, and energy, then breaking them down as they perform their respective functions. The oxygen we breathe, the food we eat, and the water we drink provide the raw materials which fuel our chemical factories. We excrete in various ways the waste products created by these complex chemical reactions.

Medicines are carbon compounds capable of intervening within our bodies to correct the malfunctions we call disease. The number of conceivable carbon compounds is, for all practical purposes, infinite, far exceeding the total number of chemical compounds of all other elements combined. Carbon atoms can combine with each other, with atoms of hydrogen, oxygen, nitrogen, sulfur, phosphorus, and many other elements. Carbon compounds can be as simple as methane, a hydrocarbon found in natural gas, or can be as complex as the nucleic acids in DNA, which contain the genetic blueprints of our species. These fundamental life molecules are composed of thousands of atoms.

The search for a new medicine always begins with a hypothesis. For reasons that may or may not turn out to be correct, the medicinal chemist has turned his attention to a particular molecule that he thinks may lead him to his goal. He then attempts to manipulate the molecule, called the lead compound, into some other molecule which will be the new drug. Normally, this lead compound has at least one carbon ring. The most basic of these is the benzene ring which has six carbon atoms and six hydrogen atoms. In addition to carbon atoms, the rings may contain one or more atoms of oxygen, nitrogen, sulfur, and other elements. These may be an integral part of the ring, or attached to the ring at various points. Most of these ring-based molecules also contain small groups of atoms which may have significant influence on the therapeutic effects of the molecule.

The manner of manipulation is up to the chemist's ingenuity. The chemist may, for example, add certain atoms or change the order of the atoms in the original compound. For some changes, the chemist may need heat, pressure, or catalysts. The chemist may even decide to react his original molecule with other organic compounds. It is the marvel of modern chemistry that an enormous number of changes can be made in a molecule; the problem is not only that of making a different, related molecule but of deciding which of the many different possible molecules one should make. Here experience, information on the biology and chemistry involved, intuition, and sheer chance all can and do play important roles.

But not all conceivable combinations of carbon and others can be made. Atoms cannot be combined at random to form new molecules. Chemistry has its rules which dictate the number and the kinds of atoms that can be attached to one another. In their work on a particular compound, medicinal chemists have an indispensable tool, the structural formula. It is, in effect, a map of the compound's chemical structure. It shows all the different atoms and combinations of atoms that make up the compound; and it shows where each part is in relation to the whole. Chemical compounds exist in three dimensions so that the reality of their components' placement, relative to each other, is more complex than can be shown in a two-dimensional diagram.

It is a major triumph of modern chemistry that chemists can now deduce the structural formula of a complex carbon compound. We now know that a group of atoms has properties that depend upon how they are connected to each other and in what order. The same atoms can be connected in many different configurations and different orders than they were originally. Each rearrangement represents a different compound which may have very different properties from another configuration of the original compound.

Once the chemist has synthesized a molecule of a particular configuration, the question arises: Is this compound any good as a medicine? Ideally we are looking for new compounds that will be:

— able to cure an incurable disease
— more effective than an existing drug
— less likely to cause side effects than existing drugs
— able to prevent the onset of a condition or disease.

But the chemist knows that for any given new compound, the chances that it will someday be a useful medicine are very slight. A rule of thumb in the pharmaceutical industry is that only one of every 10,000 compounds synthesized by medicinal chemists ever proves to be useful. At a highly productive firm like Janssen Pharmaceutica, the success ratio is less formidable — approximately one out of every 1,000 compounds — but that is still daunting.

The harsh truth is that most new compounds prepared in pharmaceutical laboratories live or are under active consideration only briefly and then die in deserved obscurity. However, pharmaceutical companies keep either a sample or a record of every compound they synthesize, just in case new knowledge or future needs should require reexamination of previously prepared compounds.

An example is provided by the molecule Retrovir (AZT). Announcement of this compound's synthesis was made in a scientific publication issued in 1964. But it was then abandoned because it showed no promise as an anti-cancer compound, the purpose for which it had been synthesized. Then in the late 1970's, it was resynthesized, on the basis of the published literature, by a Burroughs Wellcome chemist who wanted to use the compound for purely technical purposes. This made the compound available in 1984 when it was one of many compounds screened to see if it had any effect against a particular virus. Only then was it found to be the best drug against AIDS known at that time.

The task of finding useful medicines among newly synthesized compounds is like finding a needle in a haystack. Even after a promising new compound has been found, the pharmaceutical industry estimates that it takes an average of ten years to bring a new medicine from the laboratory to the patient and that it costs, on average, about $150 million.

The new compound goes first to the pharmacologist, whose job is to determine whether the compound has any properties that make it worth following up. On the one hand, the pharmacologist's nightmares are filled with images of compounds with magical medical properties that he failed to recognize and, therefore, recommended be abandoned. On the other hand, he may place an exaggerated estimate on a compound which will then undergo further intensive and expensive study, but will finally prove to be too weak in its effect or too toxic to be used.

A pharmacologist works first with a series of tests in the preclinical phase of development using simple, quick, and inexpensive tests in mice and other small animals to determine whether or not a compound has any therapeutic properties. The tests that may be made by the pharmacologist are numerous and ingenious. In any particular case, they will be selected in light of the original hypothesis that the new compound being tested has specifically new or improved properties. But the pharmacologist always has his eye open for the unexpected, since unexpected results are often the most important. Every now and then the pharmacologist will report that a new compound does show some interesting properties.

Also, at an early point, a chemical information specialist will search a computer data base that gives the formulas of all patented compounds. If the new compound turns out to be already patented, it is usually dropped from further investigation. There are two reasons for this. First, if another pharmaceutical company discovered this compound and valued it enough to patent it, then presumably that company also investigated the compound's properties. Second, it is not economical for a company to pursue development of a drug for which it is not guaranteed exclusive marketing rights. The patent guarantees that only one company will be able to sell that medicine and, hopefully, to make the profit which can be applied to future research. Of course, a company which discovers a new drug may not want to actually market it for a variety of reasons. In that case the innovator company will license some other firm to sell the drug and will receive a royalty on sales as compensation.

But the patent exists only for a limited period, after which other companies can produce that compound. Without the patent system, every new medicine would quickly be copied by companies that did not invest in the costly research and development that led to the discovery of the new drug. In such a world, there would be no incentive for pharmaceutical research and innovation. The subject of new medicines would be written about only in history books.

But what happens next to that new and unusual compound that possesses enough interesting properties to justify further research? Initially, this research will go down two paths. The first will attempt to confirm that these new properties are real by testing the new compound in larger animals. The pharmacologists who handle this stage of tests are trying to see whether the new compound is really more effective than any existing medicine or has desirable properties unavailable in existing medicine. The more species of animals in which the new compound is shown to be effective, the more likely it is that this compound will be considered as a human medicine.

The second path of investigation concerns safety, the province of the toxicologist. Initially, the toxicologist will consider short-term safety. How much of this new compound can be given without causing sickness or death? Is the therapeutic dose of the new compound far below the lethal dose? If the answer is yes, it suggests that the compound is relatively safe. But if the therapeutic dose is close to the lethal dose, there will be long and hard thought about whether it is worth continuing to work with this compound.

And what about other side effects? Does the compound tend to make different test animals more agitated, diarrhetic, apathetic, or extremely allergic? The initial short-term safety tests on animals are often done for three-month periods, and if these results are satisfactory, tests lasting a year will be carried out. Ideally the investigators would like to find medicines with no harmful side effects at all. But all past experience has shown that such hopes are illusions. All medicines have side effects in at least a few people. The trick is to find medicines which do the most good with the fewest harmful side effects.

But short-term safety is only the beginning. What about long-term effects? Will a new compound taken for years prove to be carcinogenic? Will a new compound taken during pregnancy result in malformed offspring? These are some of the questions investigated by the toxicologists, who will follow groups of animals, some receiving the research compound and some not, for two years. The animals will be meticulously inspected daily or several times a week. It is not unusual for such a two-year safety test to cost $500,000 or more.

Meanwhile, the medicinal chemist has not been idle while effectiveness and safety testing are in progress. The chemist has been concerned with what actually gives this compound its special properties. Can this molecule be changed so that it will have even better properties and be even safer than the molecule which first caused excitement and attention among the researchers?

Such investigations can spawn more new compounds for

testing. In so doing, the chemist is able to narrow his aim by focusing on the latest compound to show interesting properties. That, in turn, becomes the lead compound. At each stage the chemist is trying to find a new lead compound with properties that are even more impressive than its predecessors. The hope is that more precisely aimed molecular manipulation will result in a more encouraging compound.

People who work in pharmaceutical research and development must be capable of bearing frequent frustration and disappointment without losing interest, initiative, and enthusiasm. They soon find out that even the great majority of new compounds which seem promising on first screening sooner or later become casualties. The improvement the new compound offers over existing medicines may actually be minimal or there may be serious side effects associated with the drug. There may also be long-term side effects that reveal themselves later. All of these, and other factors, may force the decision to abandon a new compound and write off the research investment that has been spent investigating it.

But if all these challenges have been met, and if, on the basis of animal and tissue tests the new compound seems to be safe, effective, and possibly an improvement over existing medicines, then it is ready for testing in human beings. This is the most important, expensive, and delicate stage of drug testing.

These clinical trials carry the most responsibility for all concerned. It is very important that all people who participate in these trials do so voluntarily, under informed consent. All are told that they are participating in an experiment. The purposes and the nature of the experiment are explained, along with the possible gains and losses of participation. At Janssen, the first human beings who receive a new drug are frequently the staff members who have been most involved with this particular compound.

The clinical trials fall into three phases. Each is immensely complex. In Phase I, the volunteers are usually healthy young adults and the emphasis is upon safety. How much of the drug can these volunteers take without showing any harmful side effects? What are the pharmacokinetics of the drug?

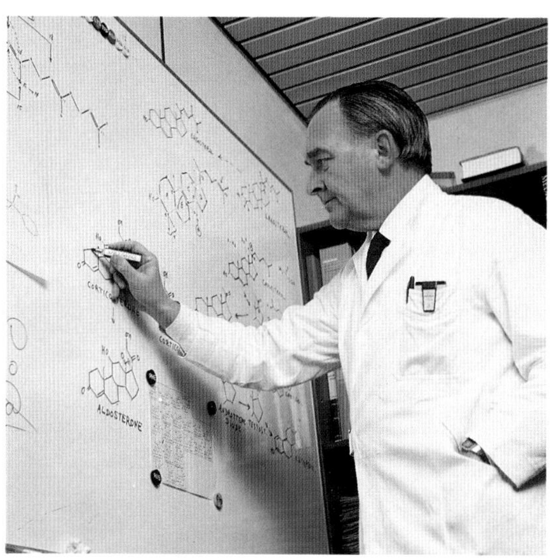

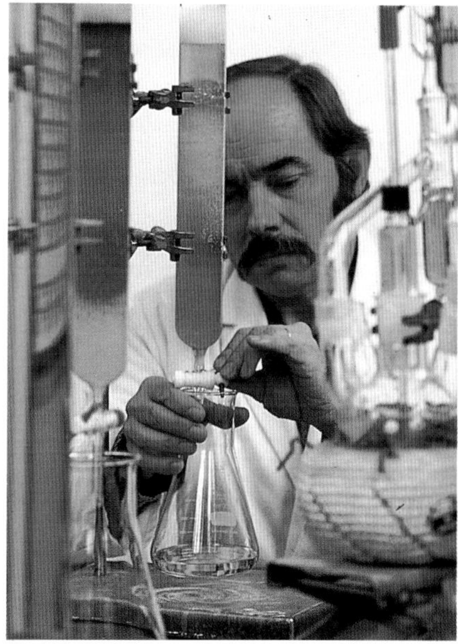

Drug development begins with an hypothesis. Molecular models and structural formulas help researchers define a compound. The medicinal chemist then seeks ways to synthesize that compound. These stages present their own set of unique challenges.

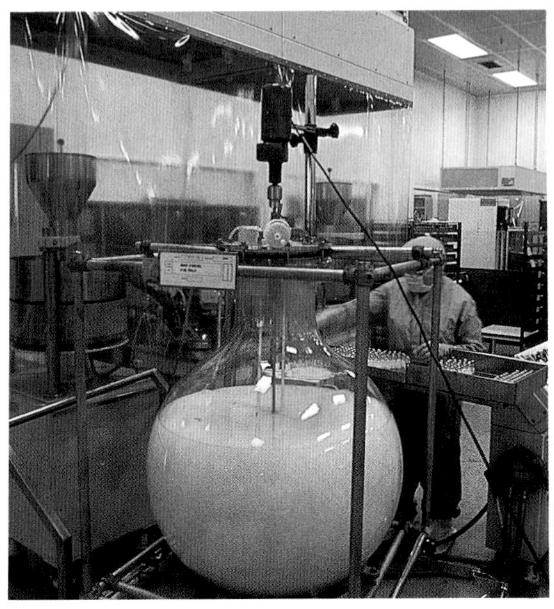

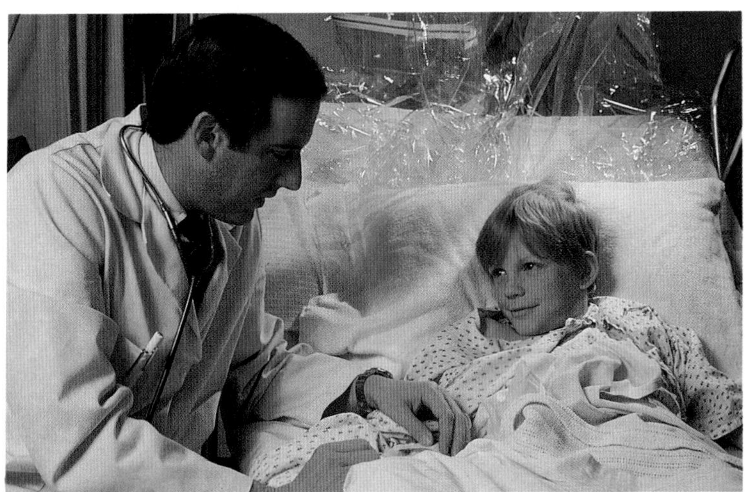

An effective way to produce large quantities of the drug must be found. Meanwhile, the drug undergoes extensive evaluations. Successful clinical trials result in a new medicine. This process takes years of individual and team efforts.

How long does the drug stay in the body? At what rate, and by what processes is it eliminated? What new compounds or metabolites are formed as the drug is broken down in the liver and other organs? What are the effects of these compounds?

Normally Phase I is conducted in a hospital where the volunteers can be constantly and closely monitored, where a large volume of medical data can be collected and where, in an emergency, all the capabilities of modern medicine can be utilized to prevent serious or lasting damage to the volunteer. Obviously, much guidance has been provided by the data collected in the numerous animal safety tests, but man is a separate species, and what is true for even a half-dozen species of other animals is not necessarily true for human beings.

In Phase II, the new drug is, for the first time, given to people with diseases or conditions against which the new medicine is aimed. The doctors involved in this trial want to know how bodies of sick people react to the new compound. How much good does the new medicine do? What are its adverse reactions in sick people versus the healthy people who took the drug in Phase I? Also there is often what is called "dose-ranging." The doctors try different doses of the drug and have their patients try the drug under different dosing schedules. This effort is to learn what quantity and under what schedule the compound will serve patients most effectively and safely. Usually, Phase II tests are run as "open trials," with both the doctors and the patients knowing which patient is getting the new drug, how much is being given, and on what schedule the patient is getting it. If the new drug successfully passes these phases, the final phase begins.

Phase III of the clinical trials is the moment of truth. These are large-scale studies enrolling groups of patients with the illness the new drug is designed to cure or alleviate. In Phase III both the safety and effectiveness of the medicine are evaluated. Such tests are normally randomized and "double blind."

In a double blind study neither the doctors directly involved nor the patients know who is actually being dosed with the drug and who is receiving a placebo, an inactive dosage that looks like the medication. In some cases, the control group may be receiving an alternate medicine already known to be safe and effective. The reason for making the test double blind is to avoid the biases that would inevitably crop up if either doctors or patients, or both, knew who was getting the drug being tested and who was not. An independent test referee is the guardian of the code indicating which patients are receiving the drug and which are getting the placebo or alternate medicine.

The choice of which patient enters what group is made by a chance mechanism, such as a table of random numbers. The objective of this randomization is to try to make sure that there has been no bias in selecting either group, no effort to put the sicker patients in the group receiving the medicine, or the less sick patients in the control group receiving the placebo, or vice versa. At the end of the trial, the code is broken and statisticians study the results. A comparison is made in terms of safety and effectiveness between the patients who received the new drug and those who received the placebo or the alternate drug. The sponsor of the clinical trials hopes that the result will show unequivocally that the new drug is relatively safe and more effective.

The Food and Drug Administration (FDA) in the United States normally requires two independent randomized double-blind studies before it will consider permitting a drug to be made widely available to hospitals and physicians. These final clinical trials represent a major investment on the part of the sponsoring company. Aside from the cost of recruiting patients and compensating doctors, the trials can take several years to provide the vast quantity of data needed to assess safety and efficacy of a new therapeutic compound.

There is no guarantee that the clinical trials will come out as hoped and expected. Often they do, but sometimes they don't. In that case, the sponsors of the new drug must resign themselves to the fact that all the money and time spent bringing the new drug to this final point have been in vain.

Just accumulating all the material required by the FDA is an expensive and time-consuming task. The drug company seeking approval for a compound is required to file a huge dossier. It contains hundreds of thick volumes with detailed statistical data on all tests done at every point in the drug's development, from the first pharmacological screening to the final clinical trials.

After filing the New Drug Application (NDA), with its vast amount of supporting documentation, the sponsors must wait for the FDA, or the comparable body in other countries, to examine the data and reach a decision. It is not unusual to wait three to five years, or even longer, before the regulatory agency either approves or rejects the drug. During this time, the regulatory agency may ask additional questions and perhaps require additional tests.

Finally, if all goes as planned, the drug is approved, and the whole complex task of making the drug widely available can begin. Physicians are informed of the efficacy and side effects of the drug in professional journals, medical symposia and conferences where doctors and experts exchange ideas, and by representatives who visit doctors to inform them about the new drug.

Successful new drugs allow a company to greatly expand its research efforts and develop drugs that combat diseases which afflict a relatively small number of people. Additionally, dividends to the stockholders will create investor confidence, an essential element to the ongoing research of the pharmaceutical company. The risks involved in drug research are obviously great. By comparison, they make wildcat exploration for oil and gas seem a safe, secure activity suitable for investment by widows and orphans! Yet without such very risky and very expensive research, there would be no progress in finding new medicines to heal the sick.

Chapter 2

THE GENESIS OF A DREAM

Every great man or woman is essentially a mystery. How did outstanding figures as diverse as Albert Einstein, Madame Curie, and the Wright Brothers emerge from such humble surroundings? This same question could be asked about Dr. Paul Janssen, one of the key shapers of world medicine and the pharmaceutical industry in the second half of the twentieth century.

Dr. Janssen's roots are in the Flemish people, inhabitants of Flanders in northern Belgium. He was born and raised in the small city of Turnhout near the Dutch border. Historically, in the Middle Ages, Flanders was known throughout Europe for its excellent cloth which was produced and sold throughout the area.

From the sixteenth to eighteenth centuries, the Flemings demonstrated great artistic and intellectual talent. Flemish artists, including Peter Paul Rubens, made major contributions to world culture. Gerardus Mercator, responsible for the Mercator projection, revolutionized mankind's understanding of the earth's geography as shown in maps. Andreas Vesalius was a pioneer of modern medical science, particularly anatomy. Simon Stevin, an engineer and mathematician, was partially responsible for the introduction of decimals in the workaday world.

Since 1800, the world has heard relatively little about the Flemish people. The area has been recurrently fought over by the French, Spanish, Dutch, German, Austrians, and English. It is a wonder that the Flemish have survived at all. This land is best known from the poignant World War I poem, "In Flanders Fields."

When Paul Janssen was born in 1926, Turnhout was a small town of about 30,000 inhabitants, with an equal number of people in the surrounding rural area who looked to it as their trading center. Turnhout was almost entirely Flemish and Roman Catholic. Large families were the norm, and the church played a major role, especially in education. The typical large family expected that some of its children would become priests and nuns. Many men joined the church, lured by the prospect of serving God, and also by the travel and adventure that might befall those chosen to become missionaries in distant lands, especially in the Belgian Congo.

Paul Janssen's grandparents gave little sign that their genes would contribute to a major shaper of scientific medicine. His paternal grandparents ran a small farm about five miles north of Turnhout. They had one girl and three boys. Of these boys, the eldest was wounded at the front in World War I and lived a long life as a small businessman. The youngest son became a priest. Constant, the middle son and father of Paul, became a physician, an extraordinary achievement given that he was a Fleming from a very poor family. But he was bright and the local farmers' organization was glad to employ him when he sought work to pay for his medical education.

Paul Janssen's maternal grandparents were the Fleerackers. His grandfather was Court Clerk in Turnhout, and his grandmother ran a school. They had 13 children, of whom Paul's mother, Margrit, was the second. With her father occupied at the courthouse and her mother busy at school, Margrit ran the family and trained to become a high school teacher. Long after his mother had died, Paul Janssen remembered her as "very bright and very tough."

Dr. Constant Janssen, who had settled in Turnhout to practice medicine, and Margrit Fleerackers were married in 1925, and on September 12, 1926, Paul Janssen was born. He had three younger sisters. One died young of tuberculous meningitis.

Dr. Constant Janssen was a general practitioner, one of

four doctors available to serve the 60,000 people in the Turnhout area. He saw patients in his office, made house calls, and did simple surgery, often on a table in the patient's home. It was a busy existence. Dr. Janssen might see 100 patients a day and work far into the night. On occasion, his sleep was interrupted to deliver a baby or tend to an emergency. Sixty years later, Paul Janssen recalled, "My father had to do his work with a bicycle, and times were very tough. He worked long hours and most days."

But Dr. Constant Janssen had another string to his bow. In the early 1920's, he had completed his medical education by taking a year's pediatric residency in Vienna. There, he met a Hungarian entrepreneur, Dr. Ladislav Richter, the only son of Gideon Richter, who had founded a pharmaceutical firm in Budapest. The firm produced pharmaceutical specialties: tonics, patent medicines, stimulants, liver and other organ extracts, and later vitamins. Dr. Richter suggested that Dr. Janssen distribute the Richter products in Belgium and neighboring Holland.

For many years the Belgian affiliate of Gideon Richter, incorporated in 1934 as Richter Products, operated from the kitchen of the Janssen home. All the work was done by the doctor and his wife. Dr. Janssen prescribed these specialties for his own patients and told other Belgian physicians and pharmacists of their value. By the late 1930's, the Richter business hired its first employees and moved from the Janssen home to a separate two-story Turnhout building. Paul Janssen recalled that the Richter enterprise seemed motivated mainly by his mother's desire for a change from cooking and household chores.

Thus from the 1930's on, Dr. Constant Janssen and his wife were in the pharmaceutical business. Over time, this wholesale pharmaceutical business prospered. It outgrew the original two stories and two more were added to accommodate the growing staff and activities. For Margrit, this business offered an interesting and profitable outlet for her energies and talents. For Constant, his combined commitments as a physician and involvement in the business made his spare time so scarce, that he gave up his medical practice at the end of the 1940's.

It is a sign of the eminence that Gideon Richter won for his pharmaceutical business that to this day the Communist government of Hungary calls its chief pharmaceutical enterprise Gideon Richter. But Gideon Richter, a Jew, was murdered by the Nazis in Budapest during World War II. After the outbreak of the war, supplies from Budapest were cut off. The Janssen company maintained the Richter name, since it enjoyed such respect in Belgium and the Netherlands, but its pharmaceutical specialties were produced by the Janssens.

As company production grew, so did the labor force and specialized machinery. In the years immediately after World War II, the business did particularly well. It was the only enterprise in Belgium capable of producing vitamins and medicines that were in demand in a population that had suffered from the hunger and disease brought on by German occupation. By 1949, the business employed over 80 workers, including a team of field representatives.

Dr. Constant Janssen, then about age 50, concerned himself with the marketing of his products. He worked with representatives throughout Belgium and the Netherlands and prepared the specific formulations of the products. Margrit, the real soul of the enterprise, supervised production, packaging, quality control, delivery, and all other concerns of a good pharmaceutical production manager.

In Belgium of the 1940's and 1950's, this was an unusual activity for a woman. Yet her ability overcame the astonishment of the community at her unladylike occupation. What was not overcome was Dr. Janssen's distaste for his wife's working, rather than staying at home to prepare his meals and cater to his wants. However, his wife's activities were essential to the success of their business. But he did establish and maintain a company policy that no married woman would be employed there, which was not unusual for the times.

Paul Janssen's education was the same as most Turnhout youngsters. From age four, he spent two years in kindergarten, followed by ten years at the St. Jozef School, a local Jesuit institution whose curriculum emphasized the humanities, particularly history, Greek, and Latin. There was little science taught in this school.

Since Belgium is inhabited by French-speaking Walloons and Dutch-speaking Flemish, Paul learned French relatively early. Along his educational path, he acquired an excellent knowledge of English and German. What most impressed his contemporaries was that he was an outstanding student and a superior athlete, excelling in such sports as soccer and tennis. He was also a superb chess player. He made some warm friendships at St. Jozef, relationships that would have important consequences in the 1960's and 1970's.

In 1943, Paul was graduated from St. Jozef at age 17. Belgium was still occupied by the Germans who, because of their heavy losses on the Russian front, needed foreign workers for their factories. Many Belgian men were forced into jobs by the German troops. Young Paul, not wanting to be a factory laborer in Belgium or Germany, preferred to seek further education.

His Jesuit uncle came to his aid. He arranged for Paul to attend the Faculté Notre Dame de la Paix, a school in the town of Namur in French-speaking southern Belgium. There the young man studied chemistry, physics, and biology. It was a secret school operating in defiance of German orders. It was composed of 12 Jesuit teachers and four students, with the latter forbidden to leave the school premises lest the Germans learn they were there. Paul Janssen thought of his Jesuit teachers in Namur as "very interesting people, very good teachers." He said, "I'm sure it's actually due to them that I became interested in chemistry and physics."

His uncle's choice of this school had been shaped by Paul Janssen's decision to become a doctor. The first two years in the school, with its heavy emphasis on science, especially chemistry, were equivalent to the first two years of a Belgian medical school.

But Janssen's life was not just school and sports. There was also a warm family life in which music and conversation played major roles. He was a good pianist and singer. In a pinch, he could play the violin, too. "There was no television, so people amused themselves every evening with discussions, singing and playing trios and quartets." He recalled there was one subject banned from conversation within the family: the subject of money. He has mused, "Looking back, I don't really know whether this was good or bad. It was perhaps good because not knowing anything about the economy, literally nothing, I was not afraid of failure. If I had known about the problems that lay ahead, I might not have started."

In 1945, with the war over, Paul Janssen left Namur and entered the University of Louvain (Leuven) to continue with his medical and chemical studies. After four years at Louvain, he moved to the University of Ghent to work with the 1938 Nobel laureate in medicine, Professor Corneille Heymans. In 1951, he received his medical doctorate, magna cum laude, from Ghent. Five years later, he received a postdoctoral degree in pharmacology from the same institution.

In the late 1940's, while at medical school, Paul Janssen decided to become involved in the pharmaceutical industry. But he did not want to simply continue his parents' business. In fact, as his education and maturity grew, he became increasingly critical of most of their products. At the University of Louvain, some medical students derided him because his family's business sold mere patent medicines, whose efficacy was not scientifically proven. "At the University, the compounds were looked down upon, and the firm had a very bad reputation, which hurt my feelings no end."

Spurred by the discovery and introduction of penicillin, streptomycin, and other "miracle drugs," the mid- to late-1940's saw the beginning of the modern pharmaceutical industry. Paul Janssen conceived the idea of his own laboratory where scientists could develop new drugs.

But to find new medicines, he would need a better idea of the present research taking place worldwide. Therefore, in 1948, before his 22nd birthday, he decided to play truant from medical school. "It was an easy year and I knew I could pass the examinations when the time came," he now says. He decided to go to the United States. He made a list of the chemistry and medical school professors he wanted to visit from New York City to Los Angeles. He had the money to pay for his sea voyage to New York, but he had little left to finance his travels. However, he found a solution for that problem.

His first stop was Manhattan's Cornell Medical School where he visited Professor Harry Gold, a well-known pharmacologist who was studying digitalis glycosides. He stayed at the YMCA, where rooms were very inexpensive. Each evening he went to the Manhattan Chess Club, where he found ardent chess fans willing to bet on a game with a youngster. He played and almost invariably won. He made enough money to meet his travel expenses for the rest of his stay. "The game usually lasted about five minutes, and I had to win four or five games an evening to make the $1.50 a day that I needed."

At Harvard, he worked for two months with Edwin Cohn, who was world famous for his research on blood fractions. At the University of Chicago, his temporary mentor was a famous pharmacologist, Carl Pfeiffer. He traveled to the California Institute of Technology for a course in biochemistry. He was received very hospitably by the professors who shared their work with this inquisitive, young scientist.

While in the United States, he also visited several pharmaceutical companies including Searle, Upjohn, and Lederle. The trip widened Janssen's professional horizons, brought him to the frontiers of medical and chemical research, and impressed upon him the economic and human wealth of the United States.

Paul Janssen observed, "One could not but be overwhelmed. The biggest difference, I remember, was the way these professors would relate to students. In Belgium, one was not supposed to speak to a professor. But in the United States, the human relations were quite simple, and, of course, that was very attractive." However, sometimes there was a shadow among these pleasant experiences. Paul Janssen recalled one distinguished American professor who, when told his visitor was from Belgium said, "I've been to Belgium. I remember Hamburg very well."

A friend recalled that one day Paul Janssen telephoned his father from the United States in great excitement. He had just seen an amazing new instrument, a Beckman ultraviolet spectrometer, which, he believed, would be invaluable for the pharmaceutical factory in Turnhout. Reluctantly, Constant Janssen agreed to buy the new instrument, though he thought it much too expensive. In time, the spectrometer arrived at the Janssen enterprise. For several years, it sat untouched in its shipping crate. After Paul Janssen had finished his studies and had gone into the business of searching for new medicines, the instrument was finally unpacked and put to use.

Having been graduated from medical school in 1951, Dr. Paul Janssen joined the Belgian Army for a mandatory two-year tour of duty. He was sent to Cologne in West Germany. He recalls, "Fortunately enough, as a physician in the Army, all I had to do was sign a piece of paper every morning, and then I was free. I could go to the University of Cologne and continue to do pharmacology and chemistry."

Cologne had been completely destroyed during World War II, but the Institute of Pharmacology was open and Professor Josef Schuller was there. "It was still possible to work. Prof. Schuller was kind enough to allow me to synthesize a few compounds and to look at them pharmacologically. It was there that I made my first compounds." Six months before his tour of duty ended, he was transferred to his hometown and again with an easy schedule, he devoted most of his time to his passion, pharmaceutical chemistry.

In mid-1953, he was discharged from the army and began his professional life. Dr. Paul Janssen recalled the beginning. "I had this idea of starting a research laboratory which in those days was a funny idea. Everybody thought it was silly, and I was only 26. They assumed I really didn't know what I was talking about. My father helped me in the sense that he gave me a loan of 50,000 Belgian francs, which was nominally $1,000 back then. It was quite a substantial amount of money in those days. In today's purchasing power, it is equal to about $5,000."

"My father said, 'Spend it, and try to do what you have in mind. But unless you succeed, you have to pay it back to me. You don't know yet how difficult it is to make money.' "

"It is very easy to criticize and I was always critical of what my parents were doing," Dr. Janssen remembered. "But now I had to make do for about three years with this money. I also had a very small laboratory in my parents' plant, and I started making compounds and screening them to get a patent."

His father gave him a small office in which to read and study, and a few feet of bench space in the tiny analytical laboratory on the fourth floor of the Richter Products building. Dr. Janssen hired two assistants, including a secretary, Andre Janssens, who still holds that job today.

The workers in the laboratory were glad to help the younger Dr. Janssen when they had a few minutes free from their normal duties. But it soon became clear that he would need more help than that.

Additionally, Dr. Paul Janssen formed a partnership with a Dutch physician turned pharmacologist whom he had met at the University of Ghent. Dr. David K. De Jongh worked for a firm called the Amsterdam Quinine Factory which had more extensive pharmacological laboratories than the Turnhout facility. Dr. Janssen would first synthesize new compounds and do simple screening tests in his own laboratory. Then he and Andre Janssens would take the compounds to Dr. De Jongh in Amsterdam who would screen them for medicinal activity. He also studied them carefully to learn more about their chemical and pharmacological properties. Often in the car to Amsterdam, Paul Janssen and Andre Janssens would pass the time playing blind chess. The game is played completely in the mind without a board or physical chessmen.

It was at De Jongh's laboratory that the "R-numbers" were born. These numbers designated a specific compound synthesized at Dr. Janssen's laboratory and "R" stood for research. Dr. De Jongh used R-numbers to distinguish Dr. Janssen's compounds from those synthesized by his company's chemists. By the spring of 1989, Janssen researchers were already working with numbers beyond R 81000. If pharmaceutical industry custom had been followed, the Janssen compounds should have been labeled with "J" numbers. Dr. Janssen could have changed the labeling at any time, but he has chosen to this day to keep this original system.

Dr. Janssen knew what he wanted — compounds that

were simple and easily made, and whose potential medicinal activities could be found in simple screening tests. He was in a hurry to find effective compounds before his limited resources were exhausted. Thinking back, he sounds amazed at his own temerity. "In 1953, I was literally ignorant. I didn't know much about medicine, chemistry or pharmacology. But in 1953, virtually everything was possible because the field was new. It was relatively easy to find new drugs."

He found the initial direction for his research in the February 1953 issue of the German professional journal *Archiv der Pharmazie* (Pharmaceutical Archives). It contained an article by a little known East German chemist, Josef Klosa, titled "Synthesis of Spasmolytic Substances." The article suggested that research in a certain family of nitrogen-containing organic compounds could probably find atropine-like compounds to prevent or lessen painful spasms of key human organs such as the stomach and the uterus.

Dr. Klosa gave detailed instructions for the preparation of these compounds. It was in this area of organic chemistry that Paul Janssen began his research. Two of his first compounds, R 33 and R 34, turned out to be compounds given in the Klosa article. Although Dr. Klosa provided initial direction, soon thereafter Janssen began synthesizing and testing new compounds and exploring areas of organic chemistry never mentioned by Dr. Klosa.

Dr. Janssen wrote Dr. Klosa to express his gratitude and to offer a gift, suggesting that the scholar might like several pounds of fresh coffee, which was scarce under the Communist regime. Dr. Klosa replied immediately. Paul Janssen could keep his coffee. What the chemist really wanted were copies of the latest textbooks in medicinal chemistry. Dr. Janssen sent the books at once.

Recalling those early days, Janssen said, "It was a matter of life or death — a matter of survival. I don't believe we really had a clear-cut strategy. We were simply doing whatever we could, and there weren't many things that we could do then. We didn't have much money and there were not many researchers. We had to make a lot of simple compounds as quickly as possible and screen them using very simple methods."

Dr. Janssen's first marketed product, R 5 (ambucetamide hydrochloride), was used to relieve menstrual distress by lessening the frequency of uterine contractions and the associated pain and discomfort. To have found a commercial drug on his fifth try was exhilarating; but he knew that it was not a major product. It was never made available in the United States, but was and still is available in Western Europe. The product could only slow down, not prevent, the exhaustion of those original 50,000 Belgian francs.

This compound was the basis of one of the first of Dr. Janssen's major scientific articles. Published in the *Journal of the American Chemical Society* in 1954, the article described the compound's preparation and properties. For those American professors who had met and helped Paul Janssen during his 1948 visit, this article must have been a sign that the bright, young researcher was maturing.

But it was R 79 (isopropamide iodide), made available as a component of combination drugs such as Combid and Darbid, that really gave the first major impetus to Dr. Janssen's career. An effective medicine against spastic colitis and similar ailments, isopropamide iodide would eventually help millions of people throughout the world.

The key element in isopropamide's fate was the Philadelphia firm of Smith Kline & French (SK&F). In the 1950's, this company was searching for promising European compounds which it could license and make available in America. A representative of the company contacted Dr. De Jongh in Amsterdam, who sent him to Turnhout. Dr. Janssen suggested that SK&F consider licensing isopropamide and gave his visitor samples to test in Philadelphia. The possibility of working with this company was extremely important because a drug accepted in the United States tended to gain greater credibility around the world.

This U.S. interest came at a critical time in Dr. Janssen's life. He badly needed to license a compound since his funds were almost exhausted. A great deal hung on the decision being made in Philadelphia. Word finally arrived that SK&F had decided against licensing isopropamide. This was shattering news.

But Dr. Janssen knew he had an effective drug and he decided he could lose nothing by taking one further step. So he spent almost all of his remaining money to fly to the United States. In Philadelphia, he met with the president of SK&F, presented the virtues of his new drug and persuaded SK&F to license and produce the drug.

This proved to be an excellent decision for both men. For Dr. Janssen, it enabled him to expand his research. For SK&F, the isopropamide-containing medicines were extensively used by doctors and helped an enormous number of patients.

As a result, Dr. Janssen hired more researchers. It soon became clear that his father's old factory, still turning out hormones, tonics, and headache remedies of old, was simply too small to contain both operations. He looked for a place to expand and soon found a large, isolated tract of land located near Turnhout in the town of Beerse. The property had once been a camp for military exercises, but in 1956, it was unused. The town of Beerse was glad to sell the land for the equivalent of eight cents a square meter, practically a giveaway price, that would be paid over a 20-year period. The one condition of sale was that Dr. Janssen had to be employing at least 150 people before the 20 years expired. When that time came, the enterprise would employ many times that number.

The first research building was completed in 1957. It was small and built very economically, but provided much more room than had been available in the Turnhout factory. The new structure was divided into four areas: a synthetic chemistry department, a pharmacology laboratory, an analytical laboratory, and two offices, one for Dr. Paul and one shared by his secretary and his accountant.

The synthetic chemistry department had three laboratories, each accommodating six chemists. At first the 30 or so researchers who had moved from Turnhout felt that they were working in very spacious quarters. But soon they were crowded as Dr. Paul hired more and more synthetic chemists and pharmacologists.

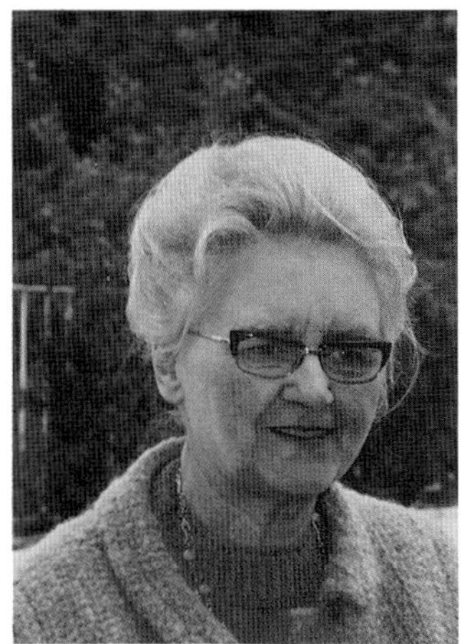

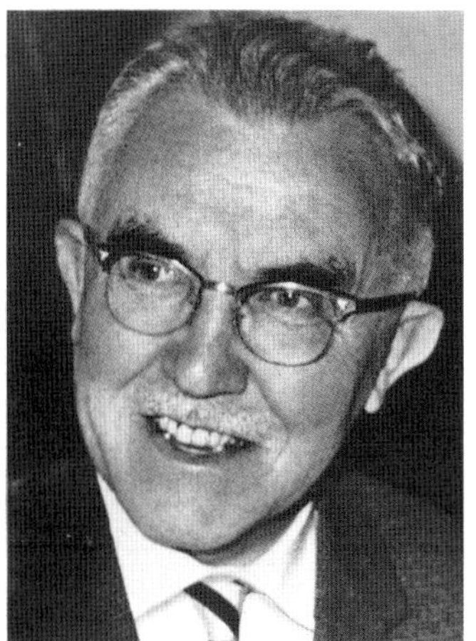

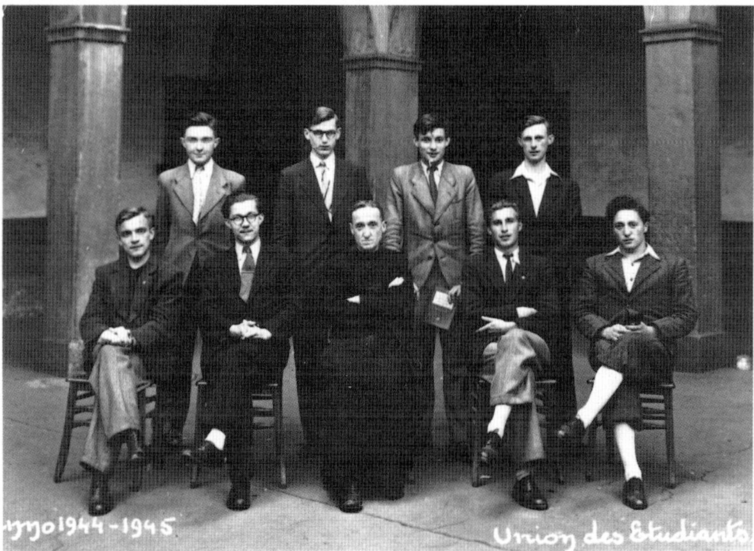

Margrit and Constant Janssen were the genesis of the Janssen pharmaceutical business. Paul Janssen's (left rear) early education and interest in the sciences shaped his decision to become a doctor.

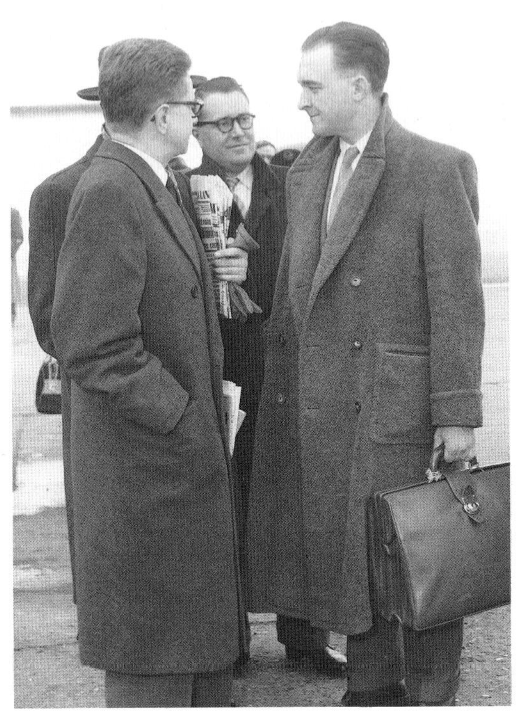

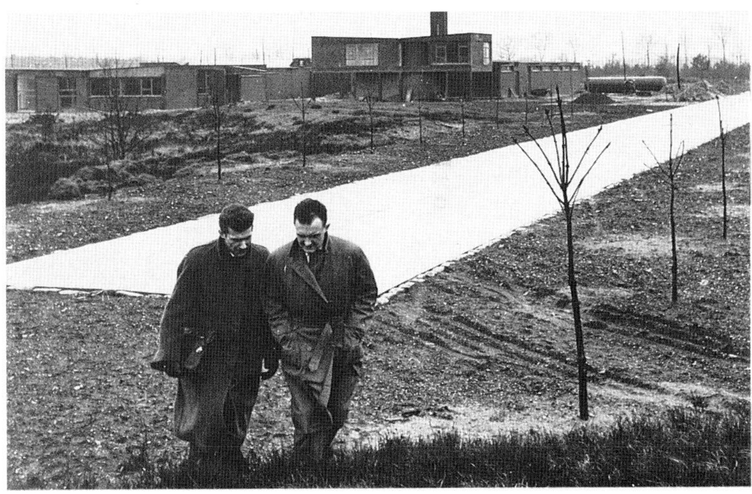

After visiting American drug companies and universities, young Paul Janssen (right) returned to Belgium to fulfill his dream. Soon after, he began to lay the foundation for his research facility.

Since Dr. Janssen's interests were in laboratory research and not in administration, he named Paul Demoen administrator of the Janssen research enterprise. Mr. Demoen recalls that he went to Beerse because it promised adventure and professional growth. Mr. Demoen, like Dr. Janssen, was about 30 years old in mid-1957, so he felt he could take a chance with this expanding company. Most others who left Turnhout for Beerse were younger, between 20 and 30 years of age.

Major discoveries were made in the first few years. Dr. Paul Janssen practiced an open-door policy, making himself accessible to any researcher. "A researcher could come directly to me if he had something to report, and I would go directly to his laboratory to follow up." He also made it a point to visit every laboratory at least once daily, and to ask the question, "What's new?" His burning ambition was to keep on top of all research, to spot promising developments early, and to assign additional researchers to work on those developments. As a result, the Janssen laboratories developed into an extremely creative and dynamic environment.

Dr. Janssen visualized an international business and he knew that English, French, and German were the required languages. Although the company was almost completely Flemish, he expected his people to speak English and German, as well as Dutch and French. He encouraged them to learn these languages in addition to performing their work in scientific research.

Dr. Janssen kept abreast of the changing knowledge in his fields of research. He reviewed scientific and medical journals, making sure that important articles were directed to appropriate researchers. When a new concept emerged in the medical field, he would find the best textbook on the subject and devote several days of intensive study to it. As one colleague put it, "He became an expert in that field, too."

From the very beginning and spanning three decades, research activities have been planned around people. Dr. Janssen did not first decide to explore an area of research and then hire experienced investigators in that field. Instead, he put researchers to work following their own interests. His assumption was, and still is, that a person doing what he or she loves to do eventually makes a valuable find.

As a result, Janssen has been the world's most prolific discoverer of drugs since 1953, producing an average of two safe and useful medicines every year. That success has continued throughout this decade despite the tightening of regulatory requirements by the FDA for all new drugs.

Dr. Janssen thought nothing of working six days a week from 6 a.m. until midnight. At first, he expected his employees to do the same and initially all did. However, several found that their marriages were threatened by long absences from home. So it was with joy that they learned that Dr. Paul had gotten engaged. As one said many years afterward, "Once he got married, he left work by 7 p.m., and so we could, too."

In 1957, Paul Janssen married Dora Arts. She was from Antwerp, and they met by a chance encounter on a train from Paris to Brussels. It was not a long courtship; and no doubt Paul put the same energy, intelligence, and charm into his relationship with Dora that he did in his work. Dora Janssen has focused her activities in art history and has collected fine art. She also travels extensively around the world. Their marriage has given them five children; Graziella, Herwig, Yasmine, Pablo, and Maroussia.

The Janssen children have pursued varied careers and interests. Graziella received her B.A. degree in journalism from the University of Houston and worked as a free-lance jounalist before returning to Belgium. Herwig has a degree in law from the University of Antwerp and is completing a Ph.D. thesis on fungal infections. He has helped develop additional indications for Janssen drugs, notably ketanserin's wound-healing properties.

Yasmine, the third of the Janssen children, received her degree in public relations, has managed the Janssen Sports Center in Beerse and has pursued her interest in equestrian sports and horse trading. Pablo studied economics at the International Business School in Holland. After serving as product director at the Janssen facility in Mexico, he joined McNeil Consumer Products Company as product director in Consumer Marketing. Maroussia is completing her studies in art history at the Université Libre de Bruxelles. She is specializing in non-European art, in particular pre-Columbian and African art.

Looking back, we see that Paul Janssen began his life's work of drug discovery in the final decade during which it was possible for an individual with very limited resources to attempt the feat of building an organization to find new drugs. Now the bureaucratic obstacles placed before new drugs make it imperative that those who dream of finding and commercializing new remedies for human ills have millions of dollars at their disposal.

At 63 years of age, Paul Janssen retains his zest for research. He is away from Beerse more often now, traveling to foreign countries to participate in World Health Organization conferences; or to involve himself in company operations in China, Nairobi, and elsewhere. But as soon as he returns to Beerse, he plunges into research, once again calling to his associates, "What's new?"

Chapter 3

FAMILY TIES

Janssen Pharmaceutica did not long remain the small business it was in the mid-1950's. Soon additional, greater successes were to expand the enterprise enormously, changing its character in some key ways as well as assuring its long-term survival. One drug that propelled such changes came in 1956 when R 1132, diphenoxylate, the first synthetic antidiarrheal, was discovered. It is known by the name of Lomotil or Reasec, depending on the country where it is used. Despite the fact that it has helped millions of people around the world, its licensing and production in the United States were the result of a bit of luck.

The executives of G.D. Searle & Co., based in Chicago, were proving skeptical about the virtues of licensing diphenoxylate, when suddenly a relative of Searle's chairman became badly diarrhetic. The new drug was given to him and the diarrhea quickly disappeared. Suitably impressed, Searle decided to license the drug and make it available in the United States.

Searle did more than just agree to license this Janssen compound. The company's executives had the insight to see that the man whose research had produced isopropamide and diphenoxylate was likely to discover other useful and salable medicines. So they made a deal with Dr. Paul Janssen. He would give Searle the right of first refusal on all compounds he produced up to R 2000. In return, they would pay him $250,000 a year as an advance against royalties.

This secure financial base accelerated research in Beerse.

Dr. Janssen slowly added new members to his research staff. It took about three years to synthesize the first 1,000 R-compounds, an average of 330 per year. It took only two years to obtain the second 1,000 R-compounds, averaging 500 per year. In the next year and a half, Janssen synthesized the third 1,000 R-compounds, which was about 670 per year. The fourth and fifth 1,000 R-compounds were each synthesized in a year's time. By the 1980's, Janssen chemists would be synthesizing 3,000 or more new compounds annually.

By the late 1950's, the research staff in Beerse had grown to about 55 workers. The production plant in Turnhout, still run by Dr. Janssen's parents, had expanded to employ about 150. The Janssen companies now included two small distribution organizations, one in the Netherlands and the other in West Germany. There was also a small export company in Belgium, called Bepharex, which distributed Janssen pharmaceuticals to other countries.

During the 1950's, as soon as a useful new compound was discovered, it was registered in Belgium and neighboring countries. That was generally completed in a short time since, in that era, only a medicine's safety had to be demonstrated. Once the required government authorizations had been obtained, Janssen's production plant would begin making the new medicine which would be distributed by Janssen Pharmaceutica and its subsidiaries in Belgium, the Netherlands, Luxembourg, and West Germany. Where possible, licenses to distribute the drug were negotiated in France, Great Britain, Sweden, and other European countries. Janssen medicines were soon helping thousands of people throughout Western Europe.

By 1957, a business manager was needed to cope with the increasing complexity and size of the Janssen organization. Dr. Janssen turned to Robert Stouthuysen, a young man who was teaching a management training program, the first in Belgian history, at the University of Louvain. He asked Mr. Stouthuysen to accept a two-day per week consultancy at Janssen to help the company deal with problems created as a result of its rapid growth. Mr. Stouthuysen was committed to the university, which expected him to work five days a week. Yet, he wanted to enter the business world and could see that Janssen had a promising future. He found a creative solution to his dilemma: on Tuesdays and Thursdays he worked in Turnhout for the Janssens, and the remaining five days of the week, he worked for the university.

Bob Stouthuysen first reported for work at Janssen Pharmaceutica in September 1957. He could hardly have come at a more propitious time. A major epidemic of Asian influenza had just hit Belgium. Doctors began prescribing vast amounts of Janssen pharmaceuticals and formulations — vitamin tablets, syrups, penicillin, streptomycin, and numerous cough and cold products. Total sales doubled in a few weeks and continued at a frantic pace from September to mid-December 1957. Individual products went out of stock and had to be replenished. The company sought to produce new products for which there was abundant demand. Production was increased by employee overtime. The chaos which reigned resulted from the absence of any careful plan for inventory control and production scheduling. So Bob Stouthuysen was given the task of putting a rational system into place.

He must have done a good job because in October 1958 he resigned his university post and accepted a full-time Janssen position. Dr. Janssen and Mr. Stouthuysen would eventually co-head Janssen Pharmaceutica, which included all research and development activity, as well as production and distribution. Now, more than 30 years after his initial employment, Mr. Stouthuysen is the president of Janssen Operations Worldwide. He still works closely with Dr. Janssen who is chairman of Janssen Research Foundation Worldwide.

Bob Stouthuysen found other internal problems in Beerse in the 1950's. The workers at the production plant had become unionized, which Dr. Constant Janssen strongly opposed. Bob Stouthuysen negotiated with the unions to develop a viable working relationship.

One union grievance was that an employee's wages were often inversely proportional to his work. Those who worked hardest usually did not take the time to exert pressure for a raise. Those who did less often discovered that if they went to

Dr. Constant Janssen and complained about their wages, he would give them a salary increase. So when Bob Stouthuysen tried to set up an orderly system of wages with defined gradations and rewards for good work, he soon came up against raucous opposition. Those who had benefited from the old system did not want to lose their privileges. Dr. Constant Janssen was appalled by the fracas that seemed to be breaking out and suggested that Stouthuysen should try to convince most of the workers that the new system was better. He did, and Dr. Constant Janssen was able to tell the unfairly privileged workers that he had no choice but to bow to the will of the majority.

But Bob Stouthuysen's most challenging problem, which took years to solve, arose from the changing mix of the company's products. Until the mid-1950s, Janssen manufactured mainly over-the-counter medicines and a few generic prescription drugs such as penicillin and streptomycin that were not protected by patents.

The remnants of Dr. Constant Janssen's distribution system were still in place and focused on the dispensing general practitioners in rural Belgium. He avoided trying to meet the needs of specialists or physicians in larger cities, where there were plenty of drug stores. Hence the business was essentially one in which Janssen representatives created personal relationships with the medical generalists.

But as the company began to produce Dr. Paul Janssen's pharmaceuticals, the old method had to change. Doctors previously ignored must now be educated and informed of the drugs. So when ambucetamide or R 5, Paul Janssen's first new chemical entity, was released, it was Belgium's top gynecologists who were first introduced to this drug. Once this specialty saw its effectiveness in preventing and easing menstrual cramps, other specialists and general practitioners would follow.

Mr. Stouthuysen soon concluded that the changing company needed highly educated and even scholarly product representatives. They could better communicate to the specialists the scientific evidence behind each new drug. When diphenoxylate, R 1132, appeared as Reasac in Belgium, it was the gastroenterologists who had to be informed. When haloperidol, R 1625, was introduced as a uniquely effective medicine for schizophrenia, it was the psychiatrists who had to be informed. But the old-line company representatives did not look kindly on the new policy that they either educate themselves to their new tasks or give way to better-informed personnel. By the late 1950's, spurred in part by additional discoveries by the Janssen research team, company representatives with more sophisticated backgrounds were finally in place.

The years 1957-1960 were fruitful for Janssen research efforts. Nine significant new drugs were discovered, including haloperidol and fentanyl whose discoveries have profoundly influenced world practice in psychiatry and anesthesia respectively. Yet Dr. Paul Janssen was not satisfied. In particular, he became increasingly disenchanted with his alliance with Searle. Although it honored its agreement and paid its annual royalty, it did not license any additional Janssen drugs after Lomotil. Even haloperidol, which received an enthusiastic reception in Europe, stirred no great ardor at Searle. In 1960 Dr. Janssen, seeing the effect that world-wide distribution would have on the growth of the company and on its ability to develop additional research projects, wanted to go international. Believing that his drugs could help many more patients, Dr. Paul Janssen began to meet with representives from other international pharmaceutical companies, seeking an alternative to his arrangement with Searle.

But such ambitions required additional reorganization within the Janssen company. So in the summer of 1960, the Janssen family turned to Frans Van den Bergh for his expertise. He was a largely self-educated, successful businessman who had no university training. Before World War II he had been general manager of a cigar company. After the war he organized his own cigar company and was highly successful with that enterprise. He was, in short, an individual of proven business competence who had excellent connections in the Belgian establishment.

During the year that followed, he acted as a financial and business consultant to Janssen Pharmaceutica. His ties with the Janssens grew stronger, as did the family's confidence in him. This permitted him to play a key role in the dramatic events that were soon to take place.

Other matters were of concern to Dr. Janssen at this time. In an interview with a Belgian magazine 25 years later, he spoke of one such issue. "My collaborators regularly asked me, 'What will happen in case we lose you?' To me that was a serious moral issue. My wife was not interested in research; she was very young and ill-prepared; she would probably have abandoned the business. In 1961 the Janssen research laboratories had 200 employees. I thought I must do something to guarantee the future of the company."

At this same time, entirely coincidentally, a major U.S. healthcare company, Johnson & Johnson, was coming to the decision that it should increase its involvement in the pharmaceutical business. Founded in 1887, this company began as a producer of surgical dressings. It soon became a leader in the field of antiseptic surgical products. In the 1920's, the company began producing the popular Band-Aid adhesive bandages, baby powder, and other essentials for the home nursery. Later it diversified into Modess and other brands of female sanitary products, as well as birth control products.

As Johnson & Johnson continued to grow, the man who had shaped the company for much of the 20th century, General Robert Wood Johnson, wrote a Credo that codified the company's socially responsible approach to conducting business. The Credo states that the company's responsibility is first to the people who use its products and services, second to its employees, third to the community and environment, and fourth to its stockholders.

Johnson & Johnson was involved in pharmaceuticals through its Ortho Pharmaceutical Company. But this company specialized in contraceptives and the parent company was looking for more general participation in the pharmaceutical market. So corporation officials began scouting in the United States and abroad to see which pharmaceutical companies might be worth acquiring. These scouts also familiarized themselves with new foreign medicines that might be worth licensing.

One such scout was Dr. William H. Lycan, an organic chemist who was director of research, a vice president, and a member of the Board of Directors of Johnson & Johnson. He first became aware of Dr. Janssen in 1957 through a pharmacologist on his staff, Dr. Theodore King, who had been a fellow student with Paul Janssen at the University of Ghent. Dr. King told his superior that if he got to northern Belgium, he should visit the Janssen research facility and meet its director.

Dr. Lycan visited Beerse, met Dr. Janssen and got along well with him. Dr. Lycan knew Janssen had an arrangement with Searle, but suspected things might change in the Janssen-Searle relationship in the future. So he continued to visit Beerse from time to time, and on one occasion, brought along Harry McKenzie.

Mr. McKenzie, who was famed in Johnson & Johnson for his marketing skills and good nature, had been named to the Johnson & Johnson Executive Committee, which made internal policy and supervised operations. In particular, he had been given the job of supervising two pharmaceutical companies the corporation had acquired in 1959. One was an American firm, McNeil Laboratories, and the other was a small Swiss firm, Cilag-Chemie. The plan had been to sell McNeil's prescription drugs internationally through Cilag, but for various reasons that was not feasible. So Mr. McKenzie found himself in need of new drugs he could license or acquire for marketing by McNeil and Cilag. In 1986 Dr. Lycan recalled his visit to Beerse with Mr. McKenzie.

"I took Harry out to meet Paul Janssen, and, of course, the inevitable happened. He was impressed, just as everybody else is impressed by Dr. Janssen. One of the elements that enters into anything said about Dr. Janssen is that he never gives you the impression of being secretive, like most of the industry. Paul, to this day, talks very frankly about what he is doing, what he wants to do, how he is doing it, and so on. He doesn't give a hoot who hears him. Now I won't say he doesn't have secrets, but at the same time, he is more open about what he is doing and how he is doing it than anybody I have ever met in the pharmaceutical industry."

Harry McKenzie was apparently captivated by what Dr. Janssen told him. Presumably he was most taken by the vista Dr. Paul Janssen drew of all the new drugs he had in his research pipeline. Dr. Lycan recalls that McKenzie was well aware that Janssen had three successful drugs available in America. So in early 1961, Johnson & Johnson decided to try to acquire the Janssen enterprise.

Harry McKenzie and Gustav Lienhard headed the Johnson & Johnson team. They traveled to Turnhout and engaged in what Dr. Lycan recalled as "a tough negotiation." Other members of the team included Norman St. Landau, the lawyer who drew up all the legal documents, and Dr. Charles F. (Jim) Kade, who was then research director at McNeil.

The Janssen negotiating team consisted of two people, Dr. Paul Janssen and Frans Van den Bergh. An agreement was reached, merging all four Janssen enterprises in Turnhout, Beerse, Holland, and West Germany with Johnson & Johnson. All Janssen stock was exchanged for Johnson & Johnson stock for an agreed amount. Dr. Janssen's father and mother retired from the business, leaving Dr. Paul as the sole family member connected with the consolidated organization that was now known as Janssen Pharmaceutica, a wholly owned subsidiary of Johnson & Johnson. The Janssen family had been paid on the same basis as the owners of McNeil and Cilag, 33 times the annual net earnings. Fundamentally, Johnson & Johnson had made an investment in the genius of Dr. Janssen and his future creativity.

Paul Janssen later said, "J&J became my insurance premium. From a selfish point of view the sale was foolish and in hindsight nothing has happened to me. But I could not have known that in 1961. What is done cannot be undone, and I did not complain. J&J did not just take over. That would have been unacceptable to me. Our independence was respected, and as long as this is a profitable business that relationship will not be altered. They do not meddle with our management, and I would not bear that." Janssen Pharmaceutica remained an enterprise completely grounded in the Flemish culture, staffed mainly by people whose language, national laws, customs, and modes of thought were very different from those of Americans. Dr. Janssen had given ultimate control of his organization to a foreign corporation headquartered in New Brunswick, New Jersey, that knew little or nothing of pharmaceutical research as Dr. Janssen understood it.

Janssen and Johnson & Johnson began what would become a long and productive relationship. Although the potentials for friction and confrontation were enormous, differences between the two were quickly resolved. But what specific factors have made this acquisition so successful?

First, the Janssen enterprise has been enormously productive and profitable. The June 1985 issue of Worldwide, a Johnson & Johnson corporate magazine, stated, "Sales of products discovered by Janssen Pharmaceutica have achieved a compound growth rate of 28 percent annually since Janssen's merger with Johnson & Johnson in 1961."

Simple arithmetic shows that over a 23-year period, a compound annual growth rate of 28 percent multiplies the base figure about 300 times. Of course, this growth figure includes sizable inflation and makes no allowance for the substantial increase of research, development, and production costs. For example, there are now over 800 people employed in R&D in Beerse against 200 in 1961. And development costs — notably the cost of clinical trials which now require many more patients and cover much longer periods than earlier — have soared since the early 1960s. Very clearly Johnson & Johnson's profits from Janssen have not risen anything like 300 times. But whatever the correct figure is for the increase of Janssen profitability over the past quarter of a century, it seems indisputable that the Janssen purchase was an act of major good judgment and foresight by Johnson & Johnson.

Second, a Johnson & Johnson tradition gives subsidiaries extensive independence so long as they perform satisfactorily. The company has about 160 subsidiaries in many different health care and related fields. Clearly over the years, Johnson & Johnson has grown accustomed to relatively different and even idiosyncratic work styles in its subsidiaries. But tolerance for diversity depends upon results. If Janssen Pharmaceutica had not been so productive and profitable over the years, it is unlikely it would have been permitted to remain today, as it was in 1961, an overwhelmingly Flemish firm, solidly rooted in its original traditions and culture and enjoying an enormous amount of autonomy.

Third, Johnson & Johnson has been fortunate in its selection of executives responsible for the Janssen operations. This began with Harry McKenzie, who participated directly in the negotiations to purchase Janssen and who was, until his death, the executive committee member in charge of Janssen. Mr. McKenzie understood the special characteristics of Dr. Janssen and his associates and followed a policy that reflected his respect for them.

As Dr. Lycan, who succeeded Mr. McKenzie as executive committee member in charge of Janssen, said, "Harry and I went there on one occasion so I could see how he was managing Janssen. Harry was doing a lot of listening and asking a lot of questions. When he disagreed with Paul, or there was an occasion for disagreement, he went at it very cautiously, effectively, and very tactfully."

Dr. Lycan supervised Janssen, Cilag, and McNeil for five-and-one-half years. He and Dr. Janssen worked well together. But Dr. Lycan, like others who would follow him, faced recurrent pressures from his superiors to tighten control over operations in Beerse, pressures he resisted. He once told Gustav Lienhard, president of Johnson & Johnson, "You cannot run that business from New Brunswick. In the first place we don't know enough legally. We also don't know enough about the customs, the medical profession, the health care system or the regulatory agency. The Janssen people do."

A fourth factor in the successful and relatively smooth collaboration between Beerse and New Brunswick was undoubtedly Frans Van den Bergh, the Chairman of Janssen Pharmaceutica. He enjoyed the confidence of both sides and could understand both points of view, a factor that helped both to accept needed compromises.

In a letter written on January 22, 1970, to Dr. William J. Haines, who had succeeded Dr. Lycan as the executive committee member to whom Janssen Pharmaceutica reported,

Mr. Van den Bergh expressed some basic concerns of both Janssen and Johnson & Johnson. He wrote, "...Janssen has been a wholly owned Johnson & Johnson affiliate for over eight years now. The Janssen staff has remained predominantly Flemish-Belgian. Since Janssen is their employer, and their professional home, and the company with which they wish to make their careers, the staff is obviously very Janssen-minded. They regard themselves first as Janssen and then as Johnson & Johnson employees, which is as it should be. ...Johnson & Johnson expects of Janssen new products, large profits and high dividends."

"This expectation has been largely fulfilled over the last few years, and apart from unforeseeable developments, will continue to be fulfilled in the next years on condition that Janssen is allowed to be itself and to continue growing as a dynamic community. This will result in more successful research, increased product development, and expansion of its production capacity to meet future requirements. In short, it must be allowed to grow in every respect."

But conflicts did arise. Harry McKenzie was interested in buying Janssen because his other two companies, Cilag and McNeil, needed products to market. But the Janssen people were unhappy at the idea that their hard-found drugs should automatically be given to other companies in the Johnson & Johnson family. Ever impatient, Dr. Janssen sometimes believed that delays in putting his drugs on the American market were the result of lack of interest by these Johnson & Johnson companies. He would have been happier if he could have organized competitions among pharmaceutical companies seeking to license his pharmaceuticals. Then, if a Johnson & Johnson company won a license, he could be certain of its interest.

But in the mid-1960's, as these struggles were being resolved, the United States was making a historic change in its drug approval mechanism. It was shifting from the era when a drug could be marketed once its safety had been shown to the era when a drug's safety and efficacy must both be proven for approval. To demonstrate efficacy, the Food and Drug Administration (FDA) in Washington, D.C., was demanding much more evidence in the way of scrupulously conducted clinical trials than it had ever demanded before.

The Janssen people found it difficult at first to adjust to this enormous change. They were still untouched in their home territory by the new winds blowing from Washington. They were accustomed to presenting evidence that under the new standards might be dismissed as anecdotal. Janssen's suspicion that delays in winning drug approval were caused by Johnson & Johnson errors or neglect was false. Also the priorities and competence of other Johnson & Johnson companies were not the same as Janssen's. The deliberately loose control by Johnson & Johnson had allowed differences to arise that were reminiscent of those among completely independent companies.

In the early 1970's, Dr. Janssen suggested, and New Brunswick agreed, that a special unit be created to expedite the approval of Janssen drugs through the FDA. Paul Janssen would fund the unit called Janssen R&D, Inc. Its key operator was Roger Aspeling. Trained as a pharmacist in South Africa, Mr. Aspeling had extensive experience in gaining drug approval for the Johnson & Johnson organization in Canada. Mr. Aspeling's counterpart in Beerse was Viviane Schuermans, who gathered information on Janssen drugs from around the world and facilitated the registration of Janssen products in different countries.

The first product submitted to the FDA by this new team was Vermox (mebendazole), R 17635, an extremely effective medicine against intestinal parasitic infections. Approval for Vermox was gained in 14 months, a highly satisfactory record. The second product was Imodium (loperamide), R 18553, an antidiarrheal drug even more potent and longer acting than Lomotil. This, too, received approval from the FDA in a comparatively short time.

Roger Aspeling and Viviane Schuermans had proved Dr. Janssen's point. Medicines could be moved through the FDA more rapidly than had been done. But such successes did not come easily. These regulatory efforts were given top priority in the Janssen organization.

This successful experiment also advanced significantly

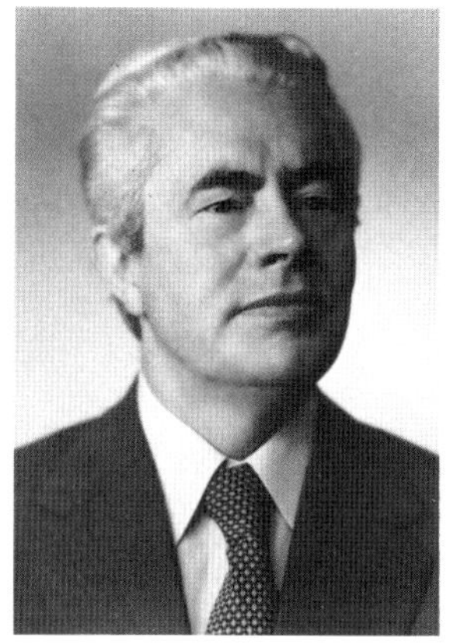

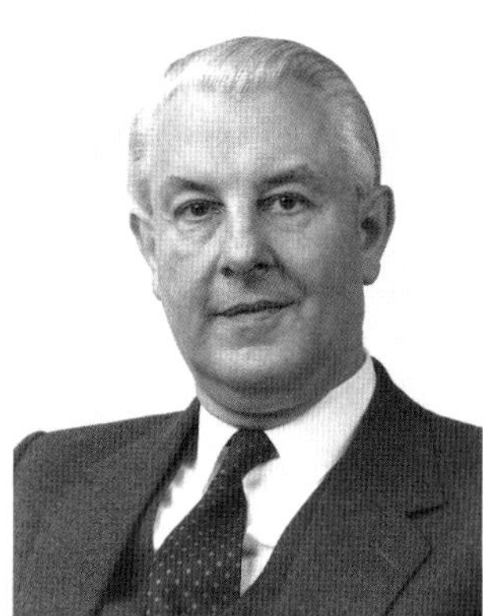

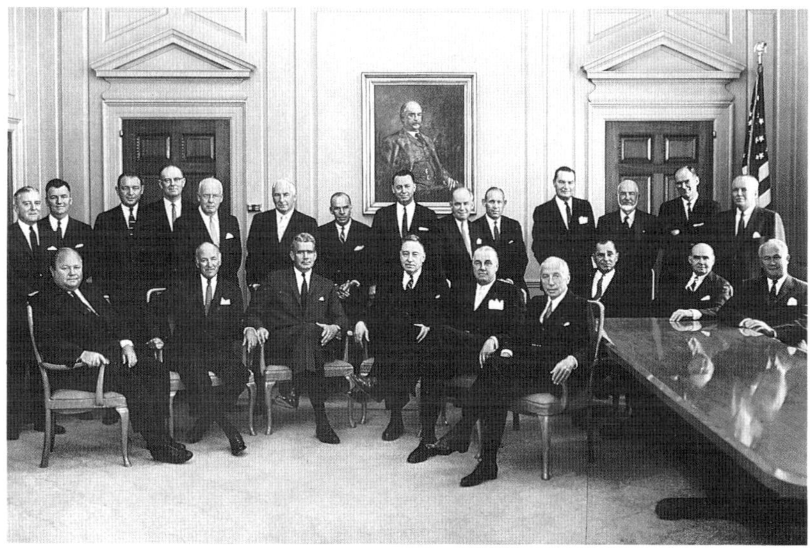

Baron Van den Bergh (upper left) and Sir Robert Stouthuysen organized the business and financial aspects of Janssen. Gustav Lienhard and Harry McKenzie (seated far right), members of the J&J Executive Committee, negotiated and brought Janssen into the family of Johnson & Johnson companies.

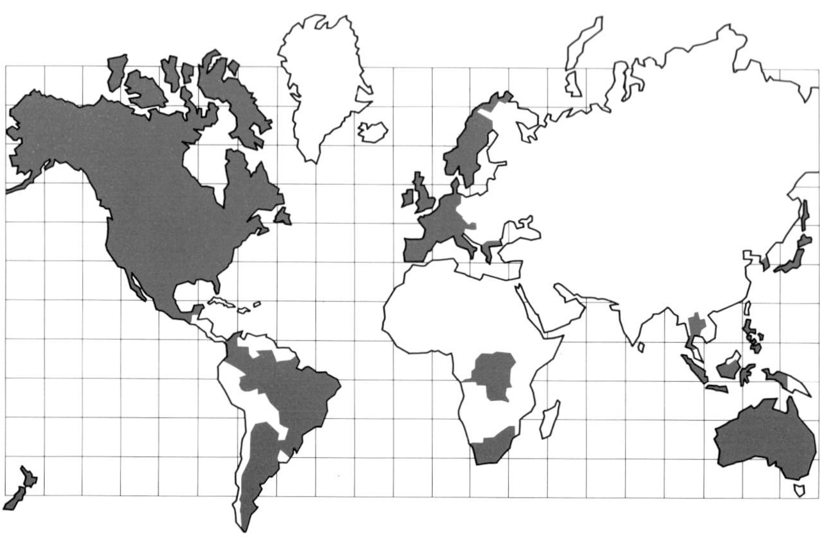

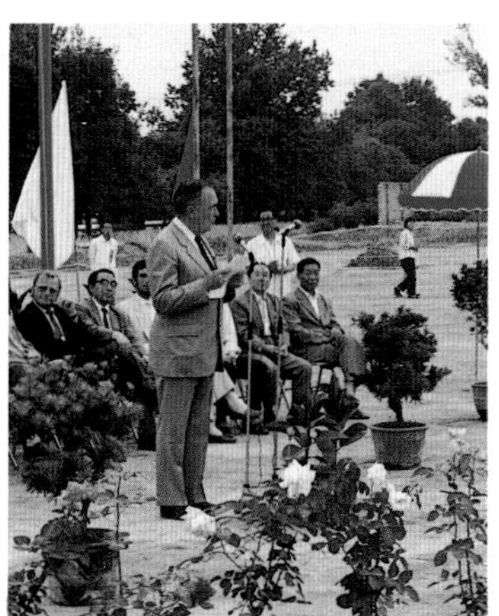

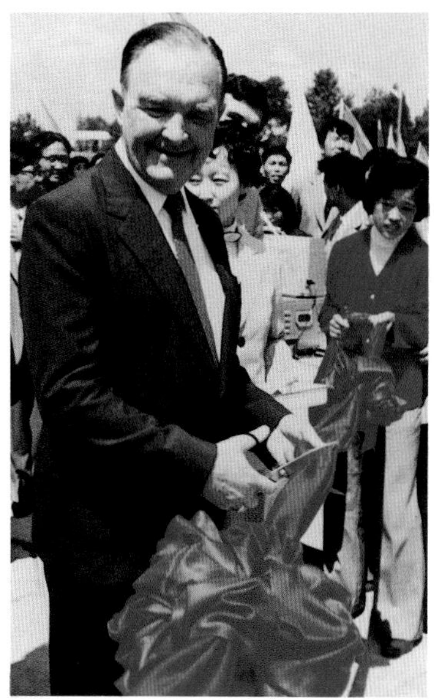

Janssen became a multinational company with affiliates in more than thirty countries. Paul Janssen recently opened one of the most interesting of the international operations in the People's Republic of China.

the realization of an old Janssen dream. Paul Janssen had treasured for years the goal his family had discussed in 1960-1961 with Frans Van den Bergh before the sale to Johnson & Johnson. It was nothing less than the creation of an international Janssen company responsible for finding new drugs, getting them registered, producing them, and selling them in as many world markets as possible. In effect Dr. Paul Janssen wanted to create a multinational company within the larger multinational company which is Johnson & Johnson.

Frans Van den Bergh stated Janssen's position clearly in a letter to Dr. William J. Haines dated February 25, 1970. It indicated the scope of responsibility that Beerse felt for their work and medicines. "We proceed from the principle that, whatever happens to the Janssen products anywhere in the world, is primarily Janssen's responsibility. Janssen should be fully involved in whatever is necessary for their worldwide development, production and availability. This responsibility results not only from the fact that Janssen is the maker and the owner of the products, but also that Janssen possesses the most know-how about them."

The international growth of Janssen accelerated, and by the late 1980's there were some 30 Janssen affiliates in as many countries. Janssen had its own production facilities in Ireland and Puerto Rico. Distribution organizations, often supplemented by independent research and development operations, were in Argentina, Australia, Austria, Brazil, Canada, China, Colombia, Denmark, France, Greece, Hong Kong, Ireland, Italy, Japan, Mexico, Puerto Rico, the Netherlands, Norway, the Philippines, Portugal, South Africa, South Korea, Spain, Sweden, Switzerland, Taiwan, Thailand, the United Kingdom, the United States, and West Germany.

These affiliates have a substantial degree of autonomy but at the same time have close links with Beerse. Five Janssen vice presidents located in Beerse supervise the foreign companies, and there is much travel to and from Beerse at both the top management and the technical levels.

One of the latest and most interesting of the international operations is in the People's Republic of China. Dr. Paul Janssen, who reads a great deal of history, has long been fascinated by the most populous nation in the world. He learned that the Chinese were producing without license some Janssen drugs for their own needs, particularly medicines against intestinal parasitic diseases and psychiatric illnesses.

In 1971, Dr. Janssen made his first of many trips to China. He began to form his own impressions of that great country and to make personal contacts. He became a friend of Dr. George Hatem, whose Chinese name was Ma Haida. Dr. Hatem, who died in 1988, played a key role in arranging medical care for the Chinese Communist armed forces during the Chinese Civil War. He also assisted in the massive reorganization of the Chinese medical care system after the Communists took power. Dr. Janssen made additional contacts with Chinese diplomats and watched with curiosity as the country experienced a variety of political and social changes. Then in 1979 he asked Joos Horsten to go to China to try to make technical and commercial contact with the Chinese pharmaceutical industry.

Mr. Horsten, who was in charge of the Janssen subsidiaries in West Germany, Italy, and Greece, was originally trained as a chemical engineer and had spent his entire career as a Janssen employee. He began as a chemical synthesist, then was put in charge of the pilot plant, which helps make the transition between small-scale and full-scale industrial production of a new compound. He became responsible for all Janssen chemical production and had a role in supervising the building of Janssen chemical facilities in Puerto Rico and Ireland. He was an international vice president who now had the obligation of creating a Janssen presence in China.

Mr. Horsten's efforts resulted in a contract with the Hanjiang Pharmaceutical Factory in Hanzhong, a pharmaceutical plant in a remote part of Shaanxi Province, in a town 300 kilometers southwest of the city of Xian. Other Western pharmaceutical companies entering China had preferred to settle near one of China's larger cities. But the Janssen group reasoned that in Shaanxi Province a foreign company was a novelty which would receive high priority from local and provincial authorities.

An agreement was reached for technical cooperation between the Hanjiang Pharmaceutical Factory and Janssen Pharmaceutica. Janssen agreed to help its partner build a chemical plant that would produce the raw material for Vermox. Janssen specialists would design the plant, assure that it had all the necessary pollution controls, provide the needed machinery, and train Chinese workers.

The plant was completed and began production in 1983. Twenty of the 120 workers came to Beerse for in-depth training in chemical manufacturing. Mr. Horsten said of this group, "The Chinese have very good theoretical backgrounds. What they lack is practical experience, and that's what we teach them here in Beerse. We found them very dedicated, and very fast learners."

The development of the plant, the first chemical factory built in China with foreign aid after Mao Tse-tung's death, provided valuable insights for the Janssen organization. They learned how to work effectively with the Chinese. By the end of 1982, before the Hanjiang plant was actually completed, Dr. Janssen and his colleagues were so satisfied with this operation that they had decided on an even larger joint venture.

They envisioned a formulation plant where various Janssen compounds would be imported from Belgium or other Janssen production centers to be processed into finished products such as tablets, creams, and syrups by the Chinese affiliate. These medicines would be made available to the Chinese people. Janssen believed this operation should be centered in Xian, the capital of Shaanxi Province. Now the idea had to be presented and accepted by the Chinese.

It took almost two-and-one-half years of negotiations, from the end of 1982 to April 1985, to reach an agreement. Mr. Horsten recalled the atmosphere of the negotiations. "For everyone involved — lawyers, financial people, technical people — China really opened a new world. You have to start from scratch for everything. We negotiated for three weeks at a time in a hotel. The meeting room was across the corridor from where we lived. Sometimes it was tough, but the Chinese in general are very friendly people to work with."

Mr. Horsten emphasizes that to do business effectively in China it is important for a Western enterprise such as Janssen to reach a consensus with its Chinese partner or partners. With such a consensus most of the dealings with the government bureaucracy can be left to the Chinese partners, who are likely to be much more effective than a foreign group acting alone. In any case, all went smoothly after the agreement, although it took until October 22, 1985, to get the business license because the contracts had to be approved by higher Chinese officials.

The final agreement provided that the new plant would manufacture 34 different formulations of 10 Janssen compounds, mainly antiparasitic and antifungal compounds, as well as drugs to combat psychotic and gastrointestinal illnesses. Design of the plant was done in Beerse by Janssen specialists. Twice during this period, a group of ten Chinese specialists came to Belgium to participate in the design and planning process.

Actual construction began in Xian on June 3, 1986, with Dr. Paul Janssen and the Vice Governor of Shaanxi, Zhang Bin, leading the ground-breaking ceremonies. Both men spoke, and Dr. Janssen surprised the audience by delivering his speech in Mandarin Chinese. The plant is now completed and production has begun.

Janssen's partners in the new plant are the central Chinese Government, the provincial government, and the Chinese pharmaceutical agency, SPA. Xian-Janssen Pharmaceutica Limited, the name of the new enterprise, has a board of directors consisting of six Belgians and six Chinese. When the plant begins operation, Janssen will have four foreigners, probably Belgians, in residence in Xian. Their positions will be general manager, technical director, finance director, and marketing director. All speak Chinese and have pharmaceutical industry experience. The position of marketing director is considered particularly crucial because the Chinese have only limited pharmaceutical marketing experience.

When finished, the Xian plant will employ 600 Chinese. Many of these will come to Belgium for training before the plant opens. The Chinese are being taught in English, which they learned before leaving for Beerse. Among those trained in Belgium were manufacturing supervisors, specialists in management, finance, marketing, clinical research and development. When the educational project is completed, the Xian plant will have a complement of trained Chinese who will know all the major fields required to produce pharmaceuticals.

The plant will also export pharmaceuticals for sale to other parts of the world. Plans to produce a limited number of generic drugs for export as well as feed additives such as antibiotics are being carefully considered.

The Chinese people will benefit immediately from a number of these "home-made" drugs. Mebendazole will treat intestinal parasitic diseases that are common throughout the country. Fungal diseases, a severe medical problem to countless people, especially in the warm climate of South China, can be addressed through Janssen antifungal medicines. Since China has the same percentage of people with schizophrenia as other countries, the neuroleptics, or anti-psychotic drugs, will be made available.

In a sense, Dr. Janssen's "patients" number in the millions. They are found on all the continents. Given the variety of Janssen medicines and their usefulness for treating a host of human ills, there are few places today where Janssen medicines are not available to cure illness, to alleviate pain, and to save lives.

Chapter 4

RING OF SUCCESS

The fundamental task to which Dr. Paul Janssen dedicated himself in 1953 was the discovery of new medicines. There are different approaches to this task and major discoveries have been made using all of them.

Some people have looked for medicinal substances existing in the natural world and have purified these substances to make drugs. The major heart medicine, digitalis, is a prime example of this approach. It is made from the dried leaf of the foxglove plant, and its medicinal properties were reported in 1785 by the British physician William Withering.

Insulin, a powerful medicine, is a hormone manufactured in the pancreas. Its role in the control of diabetes was discovered in the early 1920's by F.G. Banting, C.H. Best, and J.J.R. Macleod. Ever since then, the lives of millions of diabetics have been saved by injections of insulin derived from the pancreases of cattle and pigs. More recently an increasing amount of human insulin has been made by the methods of genetic engineering.

In the 1920's, Alexander Fleming reported his observation that a chemical he called penicillin, produced by one of the Penicillium group of fungi, had killed bacteria in a culture he was studying. It was not until the late 1930's that researchers in Britain began to study the possible use of penicillin in human medicine and the means of increasing its production.

Today, many chemicals naturally produced in the human body — interferons, interleukins, colony stimulating factors, human growth factors — are being manufactured by genetic engineering. In this technique, the genes for the manufacture of these products are transferred into the chromosomes of simple bacteria and yeasts. These transfers program the recipient cells to produce the wanted products as part of their normal metabolism. The desired products are then separated from the producing cells.

However, most drugs, including all Janssen drugs, are discovered in chemical laboratories by organic chemical synthesis. As far as we know, these medicinal compounds were never produced naturally by animal or plant organisms. Nevertheless, they are capable of exerting enormous power over the functioning of human beings, animals, and plants.

Aspirin (acetylsalicylic acid) is an excellent example of such a synthetic drug. It was originally prepared by a German chemist in 1853, but not until the end of the last century were its remarkable properties in easing pain, reducing inflammation, and lowering fevers demonstrated. Today it is probably the most widely used drug in the world.

In the first decade of this century, Paul Ehrlich and his colleagues in Germany, working with dyes that might affect the human organism, discovered a drug for treating syphilis. Ehrlich's original drug, Salvarsan (arsphenamine), and an improved drug developed later, Neo-Salvarsan (neoarsphenamine), were synthesized in a chemical laboratory. The drug was tried in numerous animals to judge its safety and efficacy before being given to people. This technique set the pattern by which the great majority of useful medicines have been found and tested before being made available to patients.

Theoretically, one might search for new medicines by synthesizing organic compounds at random, a procedure akin to that in the fable about an infinite number of monkeys pecking away at their typewriters in the hope that one of them will write Hamlet or Macbeth. But pharmaceutical companies have only finite resources that would be exhausted very quickly if they were to search for new drugs by synthesizing new compounds at random.

To avoid such activity, pharmaceutical chemists and pharmacologists generate hypotheses that guide their work. They search biological literature, intently looking for clues to the way the body works. Such clues may suggest new compounds to be synthesized to either stop a natural process which is harmful or strengthen a natural process whose weakening is producing an illness. They also search the literature of biochemistry and medicinal chemistry to find out how particular compounds affect the functioning of living organisms.

All Janssen efforts to synthesize new medicinal compounds are based on a hypothesis fundamental to most modern pharmaceutical research: The structures of organic compounds can be correlated with the effects of those compounds on the human organism. Put another way, the effects of a drug upon a human being depend upon its chemical structure. Drugs with similar structures are likely to have similar effects upon human beings. The hypothesis holds that the search for new synthetic medicines must focus on finding solutions to problems concerning the structural chemical architecture of new compounds.

A related assumption is that drugs have their impact on the body by influencing particular, specialized receptors located in the cells of relevant tissues. The receptors act like locks which can be opened by agonists for a particular receptor. In effect, an agonist is a compound that fits into a receptor like a key fits into a lock.

The receptor concept, at least as a theory, dates back to Paul Ehrlich's search for remedies against syphilis and other diseases. As an accepted scientific reality, the receptor concept rests mainly on research done in the 1960's and 1970's. It is still enormously useful and it has been particularly helpful to Janssen researchers. They, in turn, have made major contributions to our present knowledge of these receptors, their structures, and how they work.

A relatively simple example of the application of the receptor concept to discover a medicine is provided by the British pharmacologist Sir James Black, the Nobel Prize winner. He and his colleagues discovered cimetidine, the widely used anti-ulcer drug. Dr. Black had hypothesized that ulcers were caused by gastric acid in the digestive system. He also assumed that a major body chemical called histamine sets off secretion of the gastric acid when the histamine reaches the proper receptors in the stomach or duodenum.

It was already known that histamine causes many of the symptoms of allergy such as sneezing and itching. In the 1940's, scientists had discovered antihistamines which prevented, or at least eased, allergy symptoms. But these original antihistamines had no impact upon gastric acid secretion or ulcer formation.

Dr. Black suggested that there were two types of histamine receptors in the human body. One type, which he called the H_1 receptors, sets off allergic responses when histamine reaches them. These H_1 receptors, he believed, were blocked by the antihistamine drugs already known since the 1940's.

The other histamine receptor, which he called the H_2 receptor, set off gastric acid secretion when histamine reached them, and thus tended to cause ulcers. The problem was to find a compound that blocked the H_2 receptor or to find an H_2 antagonist or inhibitor. A receptor antagonist resembles somewhat the agonist, or chemical key, for the receptor. But the antagonist is sufficiently different that once it enters the receptor, the latter is jammed and prevented from working even when an agonist molecule arrives.

This meant that chemists working for Smith Kline & French, Dr. Black's employer at the time, took the histamine molecule and tried in many different ways to modify its structure. The goal was to find a molecule whose structure was close enough to the histamine molecule so that it could fit into the H_2 receptor. But this desired molecule had to be sufficiently different from histamine so that it would block the receptor and prevent it from being stimulated for some time by histamine to cause gastric acid secretion.

The search took a long and wearying effort from 1963 to the early 1970's. SK&F chemists finally found the desired H_2 blocker, cimetidine. Under the trade name Tagamet, it has helped millions of ulcer patients. Yet it must be stressed that Dr. Black and his collaborators started the search with no certainty that an H_2 receptor existed, let alone an H_2 inhibitor. There was no assurance that the desired results could be obtained even if such an inhibitor were found. It should be emphasized that even though there was a correct guiding hypothesis directing this research, it still took almost a decade to find the desired molecule.

Interestingly, he had used a similar mode of reasoning a few years earlier to discover one of the first major cardiac drugs of our time, the beta blocker Inderal (propranolol). Ironically, after that first triumph, he suggested a search for the H_2 inhibitor to the pharmaceutical firm for whom he had discovered the beta blockers. Skepticism on the part of that company and a refusal to follow his suggestions induced Dr. Black to go to work for Smith Kline & French.

In mid-1987, Dr. Black contracted with Johnson & Johnson to head an independent pharmaceutical research and development group in London. So, after many years of important contemporaneous work in drug research, Sir James Black and Dr. Janssen have become colleagues in the Johnson & Johnson family, although each would continue to work independently.

The discoveries of Dr. Paul Janssen and his colleagues have been too extensive and varied to be attributed to any one or even a few hypotheses. Yet in the early research years, Janssen concentrated on the chemical structures of the narcotic pain relievers morphine and meperidine.

Morphine has many effects upon the human organism because different parts of its chemical structure have different consequences in our bodies. So the task of the pharmaceutical chemist was to isolate the different structures within morphine that were responsible for each of that compound's properties, seeking to assure that the newly discovered drug has primarily one major effect. The basic idea was to simplify and vary those structures in different ways to produce a large variety of medicines useful for many different purposes.

The Janssen strategy was to find new molecules that were more powerful than morphine for purposes such as anesthesia, analgesia, and treatment of diarrhea. These highly specialized morphine-like drugs would have one of the desired properties of morphine, but without side effects from other, unwanted properties.

The part of the morphine molecule that Dr. Janssen saw as the key to the development of new compounds is called the piperidine ring.

As we can see from the structural formulas, even the major Janssen drugs based on the piperidine ring have many other parts and differ in varying degrees from each other.

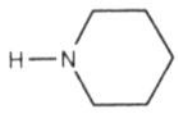

PIPERIDINE

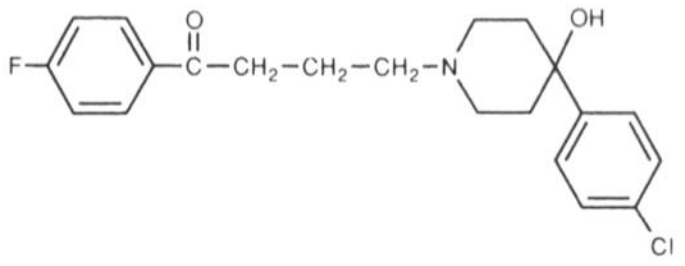

HALOPERIDOL

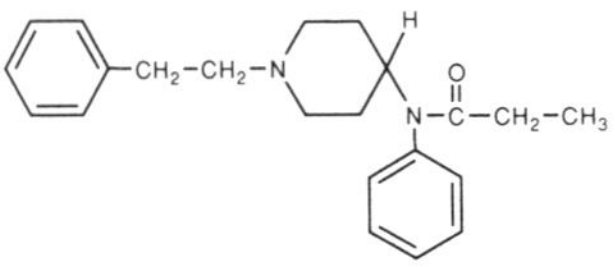

FENTANYL

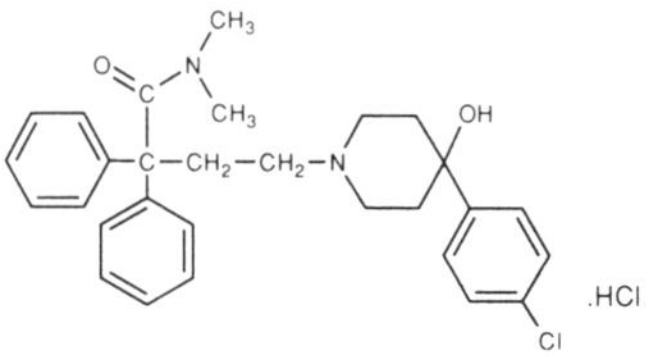

LOPERAMIDE

Haldol (haloperidol), for example, begins at the upper left fluorine(F) atom which leads to a hexagon, the benzene ring. Then proceeding further to the right we see an oxygen(O) atom on a side chain, and three CH_2 combinations, then the piperidine ring which is linked to a hydroxyl group (OH). Then farther right we have another hexagon, the benzene ring again, and finally the molecule concludes with a chlorine(Cl) atom at the very end.

Sublimaze (fentanyl), the potent anesthetic, looks roughly similar to Haldol but has important differences. Fentanyl has neither a fluorine nor a chlorine atom. It has a benzene ring to the left of the piperidine ring and one to the right, just as Haldol does. But in fentanyl there is a second nitrogen(N) atom and the right-hand benzene ring is a side chain attached to the second nitrogen atom. Finally, fentanyl does not have a hydroxyl group as Haldol does. The differences in the two structural formulas may not seem impressive but they are enough to produce two very different drugs with very different effects on the human body.

It is particularly instructive to compare Haldol closely with Imodium (loperamide). For one thing, the entire right- hand sides of both molecules are identical, including the piperidine ring with a hydroxyl group side chain, a benzene ring, and a chlorine atom. But the left-hand sides of the two molecules are very different. The left-hand side of Imodium does not have a fluorine(F) atom as Haldol does, for example, and it has two benzene rings rather than only one as in the left-hand side of Haldol. Other differences in the left-hand sides of these two compounds are visible in the accompanying diagram, p. 54.

The piperidine ring became the main theme in the early series of symphonic drug compositions. But there were also sub-themes. These sub-themes also show up in the structural formulas of Janssen drugs. There are rings with three, four, five, or six sides. Some have other sources of complexity, such as various fragments as the hydroxyl, methyl, and other substituents, as well as individual atoms strung along in linear fashion or as branches from a main path.

The results from this line of research produced a host of new drugs. Among these were Sublimaze and Imodium. Sublimaze is a powerful anesthetic agent, containing significant addictive potential, so it is treated as a narcotic. But Imodium, the concentrated essence of morphine's ability to stop diarrhea, is sold over-the-counter in many countries since essentially all of morphine's addictive power has been removed.

However, no one anticipated that the piperidine ring would lead to finding Haldol, a major antipsychotic drug, or Remivox, an important regulator of the heart rhythm. There had been no clue to either property in what was earlier known about morphine and its derivatives.

Why do Sublimaze, Imodium, Haldol, and Remivox have piperidine rings at their center? Nobody knows. But what is known is that Janssen researchers have synthesized over 81,000 compounds and a significant number of these contain the piperidine ring. They have proven to be successful drugs that address a diverse number of purposes.

In their efforts to create new drugs, Dr. Janssen and his colleagues have sought to make their compounds as simple as possible. In part, the search for simplicity has been motivated by a desire not to spend too much time following a particular clue. After all, skillful chemists following a lead can create literally thousands of new compounds that may or may not be helpful.

Beyond that, chemists must be aware of the ultimate necessity of producing new medicines in industrial quantities. It may be possible to produce a very complex compound in the test tube under ideal conditions, but be very difficult or impossible to produce that same complex drug in large quantities in the factory. So it has seemed wiser to try to produce relatively simple compounds, but of course nature and the reactions of living organisms to particular compounds determine just how simple new medicines can be.

Historically at least, a good deal of the exploratory chemistry in the Janssen research laboratory has been a matter of combining a limited number of variations of different molecules. To use the jargon of the Janssen chemists, they combine heads with tails, using a limited number of heads — compounds intended to occupy the right-hand side of the molecule — and tails — compounds intended to occupy the left-hand side of the molecule. The heads for Haldol and Imodium are identical and only their tails, or left sides, are different. By following this technique, the Janssen chemists can base much of their work on compounds whose reactions they partially know in advance and can sometimes predict.

Janssen chemists have combined far too many chemical "heads" and "tails" to think that this technique is an easy, automatic way to find valuable new drugs. In most cases, compounds developed this way are of no value, or show no potentially interesting activity. But every now and then a new compound does show some signs of doing something new.

Then begins the next intensive stage — the stage of structural optimization. Variations of the original promising compound are made and each of these variations is tested in turn. Many will show no effect or, if they show some effect, it may be weaker than that of the original "lead" compound.

Sometimes a compound will be found that has an activity similar to that of the lead compound, but stronger. It is this new molecule that becomes the object of the chemists' tinkering, and variation after variation of this new lead compound is made and tested similarly. The chemists may find a series of compounds, each stronger than the previous lead, until finally, after tens or hundreds of variations have been made, it will finally be decided that a potential drug has been found, one worthy of very extensive testing, first in animals and, if successful, then in humans.

All through this process of structural optimization, it is the structure of the lead molecule that is the guide. If we imagine that the first lead was a compound with a piperidine ring, one benzene ring, and a fluorine atom, then the second lead might be a compound with a piperidine ring, a benzene ring, a fluorine atom, and an oxygen atom. Then the chemists will make still other variations to see whether an improvement is obtained by adding additional oxygen atoms at different points in the molecule, or whether adding a chlorine or a nitrogen atom produces improvement, or if eliminating the benzene ring or adding one or two other such rings is any better, and so on.

Obviously the number of possible variations is limited only by the ingenuity of the chemists and the time they have available. The Janssen chemists, who have produced many new compounds over the years, know approximately in what directions many structural changes are likely to affect the behavior of the resulting compound. But even with experience and knowledge, there is enormous drudgery in this work of producing new compounds and testing them.

The chemists and pharmacologists must remain eternally vigilant. It is the alert mind that sees and seizes the unexpected opportunity. No one can predict when this opportunity will arise or what form it will take.

On rare occasions, researchers produce a new compound that has a completely unexpected but potentially useful effect. These occasions are very precious because the unexpected property raises the possibility that a completely new therapeutic area may be opened up by the new compound.

Dr. William H. Lycan, the Johnson & Johnson executive responsible for Janssen Pharmaceutica during most of the

1960's, believed that one of the real secrets of Dr. Paul Janssen's success was in the system he created for finding useful new drugs. Before computers were readily available to research scientists, Dr. Janssen created an analog computing system for recording every bit of information, chemical and biological, that was gathered about his compounds.

With the development of larger and more versatile digital computers, Janssen Pharmaceutica obtained state-of-the-art systems with expanded memories to hold the amounts of information about the rapidly increasing number of compounds synthesized by Janssen chemists. When some new idea or possibility arises, Janssen researchers can search their computer records for pertinent information that was previously recorded and may now be critical to current research. It can be said that Janssen researchers start work every morning with the advantage of 36 years of research available to them.

Dr. Janssen's closest aide in the collection and reporting of daily screening results from all research departments is Karel Schellekens. For many years he has provided Dr. Janssen with a second pair of eyes and ears that keep in touch with the researchers at Janssen Pharmaceutica. With a remarkable memory for numerical results, Mr. Schellekens walks through the entire research enterprise every day. He talks to the researchers and then prepares a daily summary of activities. He reviews these findings with Dr. Janssen every weekday morning at 9 a.m.

Pharmaceutical companies seek to simultaneously explore not only the possible usefulness of a compound but also its potential dangers and the frequency with which undesirable side effects manifest themselves. Promising compounds are tested against tissue cultures and in animals. If they seem acceptably safe in these tests, the compounds move closer to becoming approved drugs.

Since requirements differ from one country to another, the specific documentation used depends upon that nation's requirements. At Janssen Pharmaceutica, all major efforts in the development of compounds are recorded in an International Registration File (IRF). This compendium offers evi-

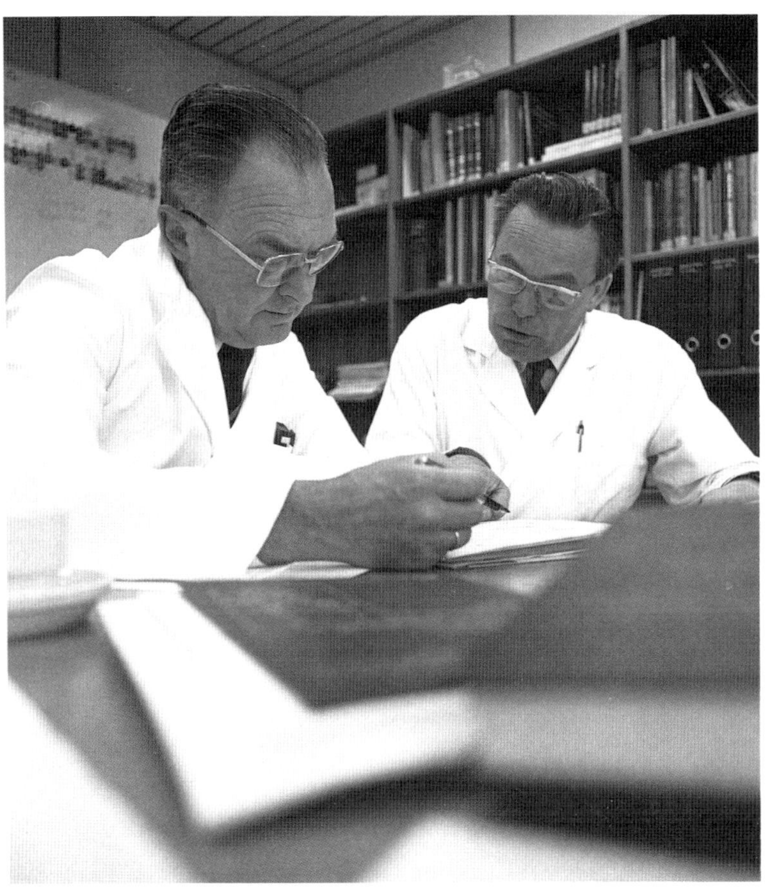

It is the alert mind that sees and seizes unexpected opportunities. Karel Schellekens's (right) daily visits to each department have provided Dr. Janssen with a second pair of eyes and ears into all current research activities.

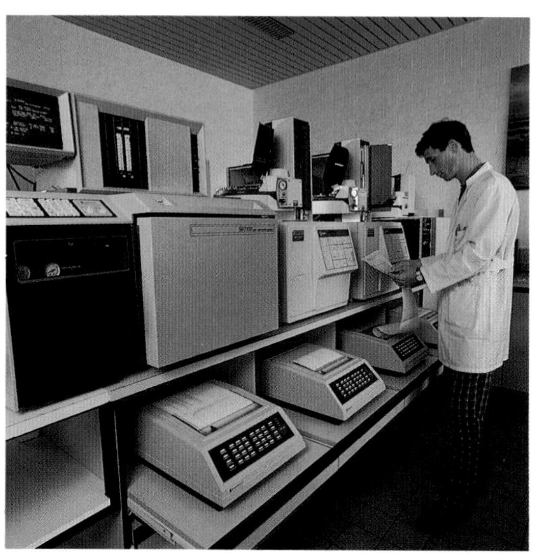

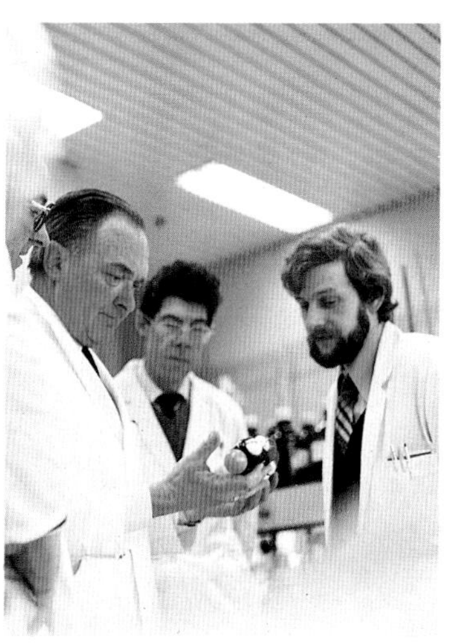

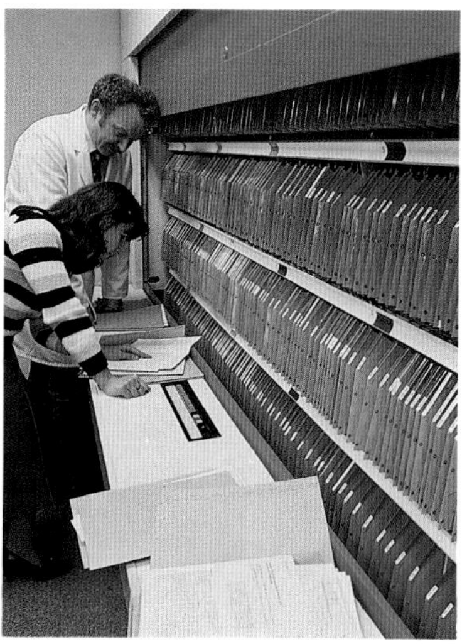

Although research relies upon complex technology, the Janssen method is basic — take a single compound like piperidine and make countless changes to its structure. Information is recorded each day, so scientists at Janssen have 36 years of previous research experience to better their chances of success.

dence on the nature of the compound, the safety and effectiveness of the drug, and the pharmaceutical forms — tablets, capsules, liquids, creams — in which it will be made.

The IRF contains the great bulk of the material that will be submitted to the regulatory authorities in different countries. The materials in each section of the IRF are geared to the requirements of the most demanding country. The IRF is arranged in a modular fashion so that each country receives exactly the same information, but in different levels of detail. Tests performed to meet the particular requirements of a country become an integral part of the IRF so that the regulatory authorities of all countries have access to the complete data bank on the drug.

At a meeting of Janssen personnel in October 1986, Viviane Schuermans, the vice president responsible for the planning, assembling, editing, distributing, and follow-up of IRFs, reported that the IRF for a new compound, cisapride, R 51619, included 1,775 volumes. Each volume weighed about 5.5 pounds, so the total weight was almost five tons. As Miss Schuermans remarked, "This IRF was sent out sequentially over several months, but even then we needed the help of professional movers and trucks." Specific information about the drug is usually incorporated into a package insert leaflet, a terse but often lengthy statement of the uses of the drug, of the main possible side effects, and of the contraindications if any. This insert is a guide to both physicians who prescribe and to patients who take medicines.

The process of scrutiny and study of a drug does not end when it is given to a patient. Physicians are encouraged to report their patients' experiences in using the new medicine, with particular emphasis on information about adverse reactions. Usually the side effects in the general population merely recapitulate what was found in the clinical trials. A sharp eye is also kept for new uses for the medicine that may arise as a drug is used by patients with combinations of ailments.

Over time, the information about the medicine expands. On the one side new, rare side effects may show up since the population taking the drug soon far exceeds the several thousand people with whom it was originally clinically tested. Any new rare side effects are added to the package insert and distributed to physicians. Very occasionally, an unknown side effect may turn out to be serious enough to justify removing the drug from the market, or restricting its use to only a limited group of patients.

Yet as more is learned about a drug, it is not uncommon to find other uses or indications for the drug. Appropriate clinical trials are held to gather evidence for these new uses. An example is the Janssen antifungal drug Nizoral (ketoconazole), R 41400. Physicians using Nizoral reported, after a time, that it seemed to cause a decline in testosterone levels.

That knowledge raised the possibility that Nizoral might have a useful effect when taken by patients suffering from cancer of the prostate. That observation initiated research to determine whether Nizoral, or some compound derived from it, might be useful against prostatic and other cancers. This effort produced a drug quite different from Nizoral which appears to be promising as a weapon against cancer of the prostate, a widespread disease among older men.

Pure chance and the alert minds of researchers are the key to finding such unexpected but welcome discoveries. The eventual outcome of such finds will only create happier and healthier lives for patients in need of these medicines.

Chapter 5

CHANGING THE FACE OF PSYCHIATRY

In November 1987, Dr. Paul Janssen was honored in Washington, D.C., by the Pharmaceutical Manufacturers Association (PMA) for his contributions to drug discovery. The pharmaceutical product singled out for particular mention was the antipsychotic drug haloperidol, better known by its brand name, Haldol. Dr. Janssen found haloperidol or R 1625 when he was 31 years old. The PMA event, occurring almost thirty years after the discovery, emphasized the continuing medical and scientific importance of the drug.

Haldol and other neuroleptics discovered in the 1950's and 1960's have been important components of a fundamental revolution in psychiatric therapy. Before the 1950's, psychiatrists had no specific effective drugs for schizophrenia, the most serious and widespread major problem affecting the mentally disturbed. Every possible expedient had been tried to help those who suffer from schizophrenia. Some were subjected to shock therapy of different sorts. In some recent decades, psychiatrists emphasized psychoanalysis and other forms of psychotherapy. Occasionally patients responded positively to these different forms of therapy. But by and large, successes were the rare exceptions.

Then within a few years, three major drugs and families of drugs were discovered that advanced drug therapy of schizophrenia. The first medicine was reserpine, an alkaloid isolated from the Indian plant Rauwolfia serpentina. Its antipsychotic effects were relatively weak and associated with severe side effects. Reserpine of Ciba-Geigy is now prescribed for lowering high blood pressure.

In December 1950, Paul Charpentier, a chemist working in the laboratories of the French pharmaceutical company, Rhône-Poulenc, synthesized chlorpromazine, known under the trade name Thorazine. This was the first of the numerous family of phenothiazine neuroleptics.

The third major breakthrough came in 1958 when Paul Janssen and his associates synthesized Haldol. It was not only highly effective in treating psychotic patients but it was the first of a completely new chemical family of drugs known as butyrophenones. At that time, most other pharmaceutical researchers were working with phenothiazines to treat psychoses, seeking to manipulate the basic chlorpromazine molecule to find new phenothiazine antipsychotic drugs.

The new antipsychotic drugs were responsible for an economic and social revolution. Haldol and other such medicines made it possible for many mentally ill people to end their antisocial behavior, to behave normally in family life, and to hold jobs. As the effectiveness of these new medicines was demonstrated, methods of caring for the mentally ill came to be questioned. Pressure from legislators and patients' rights advocates brought about the release of large numbers of psychotic patients from psychiatric hospitals under the premise that these people would receive medical supervision in their home communities.

However, this was often not the case. Many community services did not provide continuing care and medication to these patients. As a result, many psychotic individuals have become part of the large population of the urban homeless. Thus, the positive effects of the drugs that could suppress the terrible symptoms of psychosis have been partially negated by the failure of government and social policies.

While society today faces problems of this kind, research scientists in the 1960's faced the problem of developing suitable animal models for antipsychotic drugs. Normally pharmaceutical researchers expect to try their new compounds on animals which have the same or a very similar disease to the one that afflicts human beings. However, there is no animal illness model that gives a good fit for human psychoses. So how could researchers do animal testing of antipsychotic drugs?

In seeking to solve this problem, Dr. Janssen worked very closely with Karel Schellekens and Carlos Niemegeers, who has for many years been chief of pharmacology at Janssen Pharmaceutica. In 1965 they published a series of papers, "Is It Possible to Predict the Clinical Effects of Neuroleptic Drugs (Major Tranquilizers) From Animal Data?" in the scholarly German research journal *Arzneimittel - Forschung* (Medicine Research). These articles showed what tests in what animals were effective for this purpose.

The first article, dealing with tests on rats, was selected as a Citation Classic in 1986 by the major research digest, *Current Contents*. In the 21 years after publication, the Janssen-Niemegeers-Schellekens paper on rats was one of the most widely cited scientific papers in all of biological literature.

It stated, for example, that neuroleptics could produce catalepsy in rats. Similarly, most neuroleptics turned out to protect rats from normally lethal injections of chemicals such as norepinephrine. Neuroleptic drugs also inhibit altogether certain types of learned and conditioned reflexes in rats. In addition, it was noted that one of the characteristic properties of neuroleptics is that, when administered at low doses, they prevent dogs which have received the chemical apomorphine hydrochloride, a powerful emetic, from vomiting. These and other tests discussed by Janssen, Niemegeers, and Schellekens provide criteria by which researchers can decide in animal tests whether a particular compound is or is not a neuroleptic drug.

Not only are these tests useful for studying whether new drugs have neuroleptic action, but they also permit comparisons of the potency, specificity, and adverse effects potential of existing competitive neuroleptics. Some of the most extensive of such comparisons of antipsychotic drugs have been performed in the Janssen laboratories and published in various articles by Dr. Janssen and his collaborators. The basic conclusion of such comparative studies was phrased this way by Dr. Janssen:

"There are specific and aspecific neuroleptic drugs, potent neuroleptics being generally more specific than weak ones. A highly specific neuroleptic drug is one that produces no other effects unless unreasonably high doses are administered. A highly aspecific neuroleptic drug is one that possesses many other unrelated, non-neuroleptic properties at low dose levels. Haloperidol is a specific neuroleptic; chlorpromazine an aspecific one."

The discovery of Haldol began in the mid-1950's when Dr. Janssen was preoccupied with finding the strongest possible analgesic. He had achieved his first major success in 1955 with the discovery of R 875 or dextromoramide, brand named Palfium, a compound far more powerful than morphine. That discovery had the incidental effect of bringing Dr. Janssen international fame. Newspaper editors were apparently captivated by the idea of a pain medication more effective per unit weight than morphine.

This happened because a physician reported to a scientific meeting in Paris on the results of his experiments with Palfium. Unknown to the physician, there was a newspaper reporter in the audience who wrote a sensational story. His article made the front page of his newspaper. Versions of that story soon appeared in other Paris newspapers. One French magazine went so far as to print an article hailing Dr. Janssen as a young genius.

When Belgian newspaper editors read what the Paris papers had printed, they went looking for Dr. Janssen. Some were annoyed that he had not given the "scoop" to newspapers in his native Belgium. Reporters arrived at the Janssen factory, clamoring for statements from Dr. Janssen.

But Dr. Janssen was in the United States on business. His parents phoned and told him of the excitment. He came home as soon as possible and held a press conference. There had been no intention to seek publicity for Palfium. The physician who reported to the Paris meeting had thought that only researchers were present. Nonetheless, the media had begun to follow the Janssen work.

Dr. Janssen was not convinced that Palfium was the strongest and safest analgesic possible. Ideally, he wanted an analgesic without any addiction potential. For a second try at that goal, he began working with variations of the analgesic meperidine, or pethidine, a synthetic derivative of morphine, which is often called Demerol in the United States.

Meperidine had been synthesized in 1939 and was widely used even though it is only about one-tenth as powerful a pain killer, per unit weight, as morphine. The Janssen researchers decided that meperidine was a poor analgesic because it could not easily penetrate the central nervous system. It is what chemists call "too hydrophilic," that is, water loving, or soluble in water. What was needed was a meperidine derivative that could penetrate the blood-brain barrier more easily because it is more lipophilic or fat soluble.

There was another concern in Dr. Janssen's mind at this time. Bicycle racing is a very popular sport in Belgium, and as in other countries, some Belgian bicycle racers used amphetamines to "pep" themselves up. Chronic amphetamine abusers among these racers exhibited symptoms almost clinically indistinguishable from paranoid schizophrenia. Dr. Janssen's thoughts turned to the possibility of finding an amphetamine antagonist that might relieve or cure the disease suffered by the chronic amphetamine abusers.

To get a meperidine derivative that was fat soluble, the Janssen chemists replaced the methyl group (CH_3) at the extreme left of the meperidine molecule with a benzene ring. This meperidine derivative had stronger analgesic action, presumably because its increased fat solubility permitted better penetration of the nervous system through the blood-brain barrier.

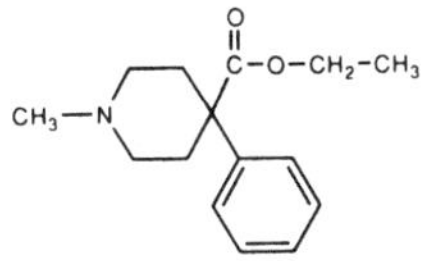

MEPERIDINE

The chemists knew that more than fat solubility was required for a stronger analgesic. The compound would have to bind with a receptor, a consideration which raised the question of how well the modified meperidine might fit. Then, between the benzene ring at the left and the nitrogen(N) vertex of the piperidine ring at the center, they inserted a C=O combination and two CH_2 groups. There were now three carbon atoms between the benzene ring and the piperidine ring. The origin of this variation may have been connected with the fact that the piperidine ring has an almost identical side chain. This new compound, R 951, showed a distinct increase in analgesic power.

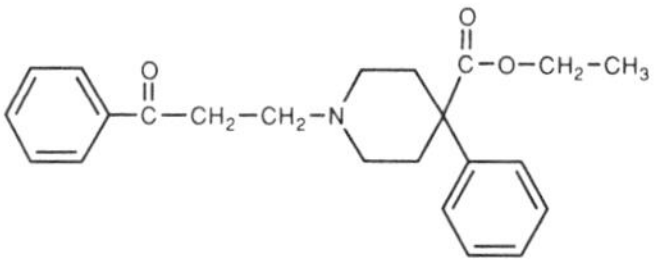

R 951

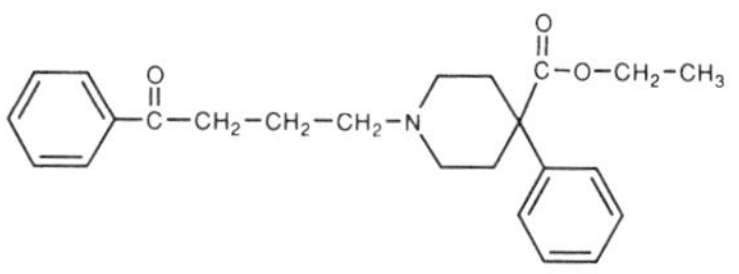

R 1187

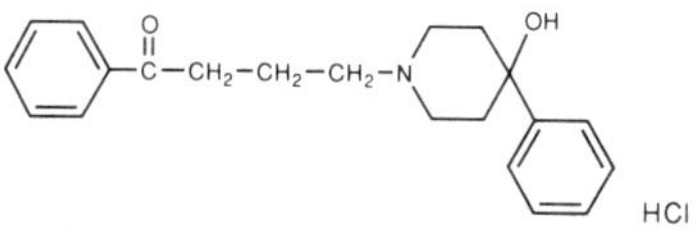

R 1472

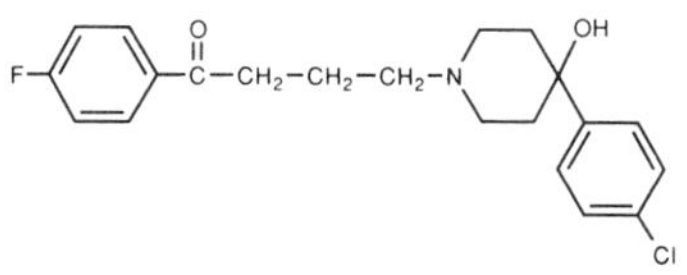

HALOPERIDOL

When four carbon atoms were inserted between the benzene ring and the nitrogen atom, however, the resultant compound, R 1187, had less analgesic power than R 951. Clearly the chemists had made the distance between the benzene ring and the nitrogen atom too large for the resulting compound to fit into the pain receptor, as needed in order to gain the desired goal of maximum pain relief. The Janssen experimenters noted, however, that when a dose of R 1187 was injected into some mice, the mice displayed unexpected behavior after first exhibiting expected behavior. First, the mice became agitated, showing morphine-like excitement. The pupils of their eyes widened to their maximum extent and they became insensitive to various unpleasant stimuli. These were all expected effects of morphine and morphine derivatives, so they caused no special stir.

But then the mice became progressively calm, sedated, and slightly cataleptic. This was unexpected behavior that had never been seen before with a morphine derivative. It was a clue to a potential new drug effect that might have possible benefit for human beings. Further tests soon revealed that the new drug effect being seen was characteristic of neuroleptic drugs such as chlorpromazine.

R 1187, being intermediate between an analgesic and a new neuroleptic, was not itself of interest except as a starting point for trying to find compounds which might show the new effect more strongly without any analgesic property. Suddenly the job of the chemists had changed dramatically. Originally they were looking for a stronger analgesic. Now they wanted a derivative of R 1187 which had no analgesic properties but had much stronger capability to evoke the calming, sedating, and catalepsy-precipitating properties which had shown up so unexpectedly.

The chemists and pharmacologists also realized that the new compound might lead them to an amphetamine inhibitor which could be used against the disease caused by chronic amphetamine abuse. The calming and sedating properties of R 1187 are, of course, those of a neuroleptic drug, and the Janssen researchers understood full well that they had enjoyed a stroke of good fortune. In looking for a stronger analgesic, their research path had unexpectedly disclosed the possibility of finding a powerful neuroleptic. This now became a paramount goal. The new class of neuroleptic drugs became known as butyrophenones.

The new quest focused on finding a better neuroleptic by making various changes in the molecule of R 1187. This was done and finally R 1472 was found. Like R 1187, it had four carbon atoms between the benzene ring and the nitrogen.

But unlike R 1187, R 1472 had a hydroxyl group as a

side chain to the right of the piperidine ring. It replaced an ethoxycarbonyl group, a complex group of carbon, hydrogen, and oxygen atoms, that had occupied the corresponding position in meperidine. It quickly became clear that this substitution had produced a new compound, R 1472, that was another major step forward. It no longer had any analgesic effects, but instead was a pure neuroleptic.

However R 1472 was useless for practical administration to patients because the body was able to break it down very quickly. The problem now was how to change R 1472 so it would last longer and yet retain or, if possible, even increase its neuroleptic action. Many new compounds were synthesized in this search. The most powerful and active of these compounds turned out to be Haldol, R 1625.

In Haldol, a direct descendant of R 1472, the original problem of excessively rapid excretion was met by two changes. Chemically, these changes protected the compound against rapid hydroxylation or metabolic breakdown in the body which would permit the metabolized compounds to dissolve in water and be excreted by the urine. The two changes involved putting a fluorine atom at one end of the compound and a chlorine atom at the other, both replacing hydrogen atoms that had been at those points in R 1472.

Fluorine and chlorine, both members of the halogen series, share the common property of impeding a compound's rapid metabolic breakdown in the body. Fluorine did more. It actually increased Haldol's biological activity, a fact shown when either chlorine or bromine, another halogen, was substituted for the fluorine. The compounds resulting from these two substitutions had less neuroleptic activity than Haldol. Additionally Haldol turned out to be a strong amphetamine antagonist.

Dr. Janssen spoke of the considerations which caused him to select Haldol of all the neuroleptic compounds to be tested clinically on patients. "R 1625, or haloperidol, was by far the most active neuroleptic drug known in 1958. It was many times more potent than chlorpromazine, was both faster- and longer-acting. It was as potent orally as parenterally, and was chemically pure, soluble, and stable in aqueous solution.

"It was almost devoid of the antiadrenergic and other autonomic effects of chlorpromazine, had a more favorable safety ratio, and was surprisingly well tolerated when given chronically to laboratory animals. All these findings convinced us that we had a drug in our hands that would probably produce chlorpromazine-like effects in the clinic, but was likely to do so at doses only one-fiftieth or one-hundredth as large as chlorpromazine."

The first clinical trials were conducted in the psychiatric clinic at the University of Liege. Two psychiatrists participated in this first trial. Both recalled the amazing transformation of the psychiatric ward as the patients received Haldol intravenously. The usual disorderly, noisy ward was transformed through the calming effects of Haldol. By October 1958, the doctors involved delivered a public report telling of their experience and declaring that Haldol was the drug of choice in the emergency treatment of psychiatric agitation, regardless of the cause of that agitation.

After this successful experiment, more clinical trials were organized in most of the countries of Western Europe. In September 1959 a group of 41 psychiatric specialists from eleven European countries met in Beerse to present 17 papers discussing their experiences using Haldol. What emerged was that a major useful new drug had been added to the armamentarium against psychotic illness.

Particularly impressive was one paper by a team headed by Dr. Jean Delay from the Sainte Anne Clinic in Paris where chlorpromazine had originally been tested. Years before his Haldol trial, Dr. Delay's report on chlorpromazine had been the first powerful boost that drug had received. Dr. Delay's 1959 report declared that the therapeutic results he and his colleagues had observed with Haldol were superior to those obtained from any other neuroleptic available at the time, a polite way of saying that Haldol was a better neuroleptic than chlorpromazine.

A month after this symposium, Haldol became generally available for physicians in Belgium and within two years Haldol was available and being widely prescribed in most Western European countries. Within a period of three years after

Dr. Janssen's decision that Haldol was the best of the neuroleptic compounds he had found, it had been clinically tested and made available to patients in most of Western Europe.

Even after neuroleptic drugs like Haldol were approved, obstacles existed that blocked these useful medicines from being widely used. Several factors created these barriers. First, the arrival of neuroleptic drugs was entirely unexpected. Moreover, they produced such drastic behavioral changes that most psychiatrists initially viewed them with disbelief, suspicion, and even hostility. Some simply could not believe that such a radical transformation of their psychotic patients could be obtained merely by administering a drug. Others assumed that drugs which produced such miraculous results must be so powerful that they would generate terrible side effects.

Second, as with all drugs, the new neuroleptics, including Haldol, did have undesirable side effects. They could produce symptoms similar to those of Parkinson's disease: palsy-like tremors, muscular contortions or rigidity. But these can usually be reversed by stopping treatment or administering drugs that tend to end such symptoms. Worst of all, on rare occasions a patient may develop tardive dyskinesia, an ailment characterized by irreversible rhythmical involuntary movements of tongue, face, mouth, or jaw. But such symptoms had been observed and described even before the use of neuroleptics.

Third, as these side effects emerged, they strengthened the forces that opposed the wide use of these new drugs. But most of the opposition was worn down as it became clear that the benefits of these new drugs far exceeded the risks. The extent of the victory is indicated by the fact that in the late 1950's and early 1960's patients on Haldol consumed only a few million or a few tens of millions of 3-mg doses a year. In 1969 consumption was up to 753 million 3-mg doses.

Even after the discovery of Haldol, Janssen researchers have sought better drugs against psychosis. For many years, they explored the properties of drugs derived from Haldol. Later, as new scientific information on the brain accumulated and suggested new approaches, other chemical families and approaches were explored. That research, and the research of other scientists, has generated more than 11,000 scientific papers on haloperidol.

The new goal for the Janssen researchers was to find derivatives of Haldol which would be simultaneously more effective, quicker acting, and yet produce fewer harmful side effects than the original drug. Trifluperidol, R 2498, for example produces therapeutic results similar to Haldol using doses only one-half or one-third as large. In controlled clinical trials, it was shown to be superior to phenothiazines when given to autistic schizophrenic patients.

Even more potent are benperidol, R 4584, and spiperone, R 5147, which are therapeutic at a dose only about one-tenth as large as that of Haldol. Both are useful in the treatment of alcohol withdrawal. Benperidol improves sleep in psychotic patients and inhibits aberrant sexual behavior, while spiperone is remarkably effective in treating many drug-resistant chronic schizophrenics. These compounds are used in various European countries and Japan but were never introduced in the United States.

Only two members of the Janssen neuroleptic drug family synthesized after the Haldol breakthrough have been approved in the United States for use with human beings. They are Orap, R 6238, whose generic name is pimozide, and Inapsine, R 4749, whose generic name is droperidol. Orap was synthesized first in 1963 and is the original member of a new family of compounds derived from the butyrophenones, the diphenylbutyl piperidines. This was developed in the United States as an orphan drug, a drug needed by such a relatively small number of patients that ordinary commercial development would never be economical.

Orap's suggested use is for Gilles de la Tourette's disease, a very distressing neurological disease. The sufferer continually makes jerky movements and shouts exclamations, sometimes obscene and profane. The victim with Tourette's disease cannot control these muscular and voiced tics, and as may be imagined, the life of such people is very difficult. Frequently Tourette's disease may be controlled by use of Haldol and it is often employed for this purpose by neurologists and other physicians. But when Tourette's disease proves recalcitrant to the action of Haldol and similar medicines, Orap is available.

In the Haldol family of drugs, sedation is of primary importance. This is the key which helps us understand how Haldol and related neuroleptics work. But to explore the mechanism by which Haldol works, we must turn to the brain and become acquainted with the concepts of neurotransmitters and their receptors.

Recent decades have shown that the brain is a vast mechanism in which a multitude of communications are always being transmitted by substances made in the neurons, the basic brain cells. These substances, the neurotransmitters, carry different messages from neuron to neuron, and at any moment each neuron is the target of numerous messages being conveyed to it by many different neurotransmitters from many different neurons.

Some of the neurotransmitters have been identified. An important one is dopamine, which seems to send messages resulting in excitement and movement. Thus, agitated psychotics and victims of Tourette's disease seem to have an excess of dopamine coursing through their neurons.

On the other hand, sufferers from Parkinson's disease, in which lethargy is a frequent symptom, seem to have an inadequate amount of dopamine in their brains. The latter fact is attested by the use of a precursor of dopamine, the drug L-dopa, as a frequently effective temporary palliative of Parkinson's disease.

These considerations suggest that Haldol and drugs like it do their work by inhibiting dopamine in the brains of people who have an excess of the chemical. Another way of expressing the same idea is to say that Haldol and related drugs are dopamine antagonists.

This has essentially been proven by brilliant research in the 1970's, much of it done by Janssen researchers employing formulations of Haldol and spiperone made radioactive with tritium, the form of hydrogen which has two extra neutrons in its nucleus. Tritium-labeled Haldol and spiperone have permitted scientists to trace the locations and movements of different specific drugs in the brain. The result of that research is the conclusion that there is a so-called D_2 receptor, one of two dopamine receptors in the brain, and it is to that receptor that Haldol and related drugs attach themselves when doing their work against excessive agitation in psychotics and victims of Tourette's disease.

Presumably by this attachment, the Haldol family of drugs impedes the transmission of dopamine from neuron to neuron, thus offsetting the excessive supply of dopamine. Aside from helping to explain how Haldol and related drugs work in the brain, this research has shown the importance of Janssen compounds as tools for scientific research aimed at understanding how the brain and its complex system of neurotransmitters and receptors work.

Janssen's tritium-labeled spiperone, represented by the symbols ^{3}H-spiperone, also played a major role in the discovery of the serotonin_2 receptor, as explained by Janssen researchers in 1986: "When studying ^{3}H-spiperone binding *in vivo*, we observed a more rapid decline of labeling in the rat frontal cortex than in the striatum. This suggested to us the occurrence of different dopamine receptors in the two brain areas. Starting with this wrong hypothesis, we decided to look more carefully at ^{3}H-spiperone binding in the frontal cortex. Soon, it became evident that in this brain region, serotonin agonists and antagonists were much more active displacers of ^{3}H-spiperone binding than dopamine antagonists.... Moreover, the affinity of numerous drugs for ^{3}H-spiperone binding in the frontal cortex was found to correlate well with the drug potency to antagonize tryptamine-induced clonic seizures in rats ... and serotonin-induced contractions in rat caudal artery ... Subsequently, the site labeled by ^{3}H-spiperone in the frontal cortex was termed serotonin 5-HT_2 or S_2-receptor.

"The work on ^{3}H-spiperone binding in the frontal cortex has provided a great impetus to search for new serotonin antagonists and has increased the understanding of the functional role of serotonin and its receptor."

By broadening our understanding of the brain and its neurotransmitter receptor system, this basic research made possible numerous other important drug discoveries. Several of these were discovered by Janssen researchers in the late 1970's and the 1980's, included ketanserin, R 41468; ritanserin, R 55667; and risperidone, R 64766. All of these work in part or in whole because they are S_2 antagonists. The techniques Janssen researchers used to find their serotonin antagonists were essentially variants of the heads and tails combination techniques. In the case of the serotonin antagonists, the researchers produced a series of chemical fragments which were then combined with each other in different orders and combinations.

Since the brains of animals have many similarities to those of human beings, it is not surprising that Haldol-related drugs are also widely used in veterinary medicine and for the management of large wild animals when they must be captured or immobilized. These drugs are used to transfer wild animals from one animal preserve which is overpopulated to another which is better able to support a larger population.

Zoo keepers have found that captive gorillas, chimpanzees, and orangutans, which drink milk containing Inapsine (droperidol), become cataleptic from the medication within a few minutes. Then these huge, normally intractable and dangerous animals can be handled for diagnostic tests or surgery.

Other Janssen neuroleptics are widely used for tranquilizing animals of economic importance. These drugs include fluanisone, R 2028, for poultry and azaperone, R 1929, a tranquilizer for pigs. When moved to market, pigs can become very aggressive and fight with each other. Azaperone calms them and prevents the loss of weight that would occur from fighting.

Meanwhile, Janssen faced another hurdle with Haldol in the United States, where it did not become available until the mid-1960's and did not receive a patent until 1969. It had already been widely available for five to seven years in Western Europe. Janssen still had an agreement with G.D. Searle & Co. that had been made in the 1950's. That agreement gave Searle the right of first refusal for the United States on all new Janssen compounds from R 1001 to R 2000. Since

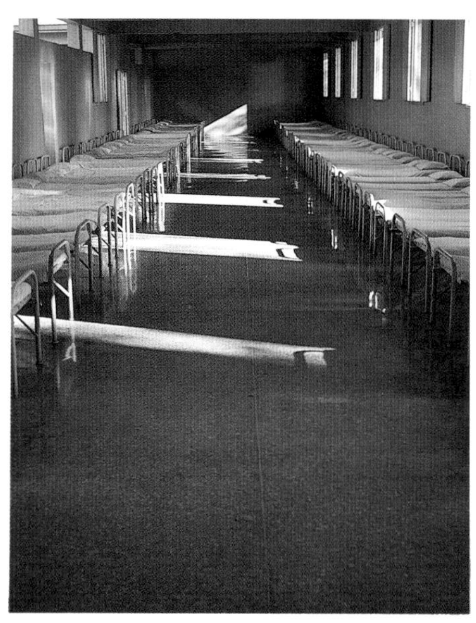

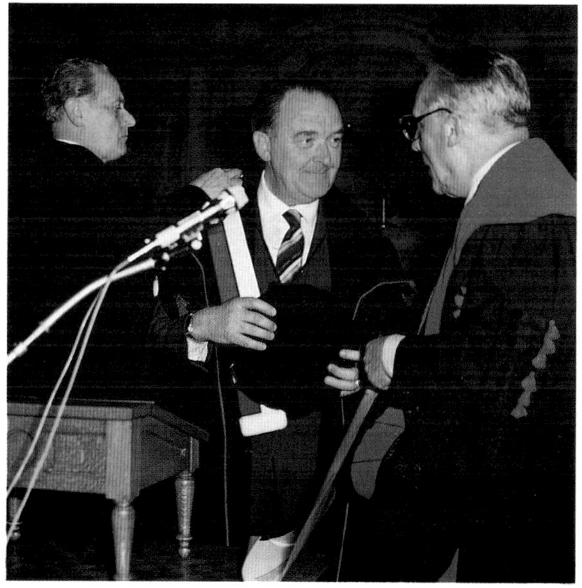

Haldol, and other such medicines, changed the social and economic face of society. Patients in mental institutions could be medicated at home and were mainstreamed into the community. The scientific world has honored Paul Janssen for his contribution to this revolution in psychiatric therapy.

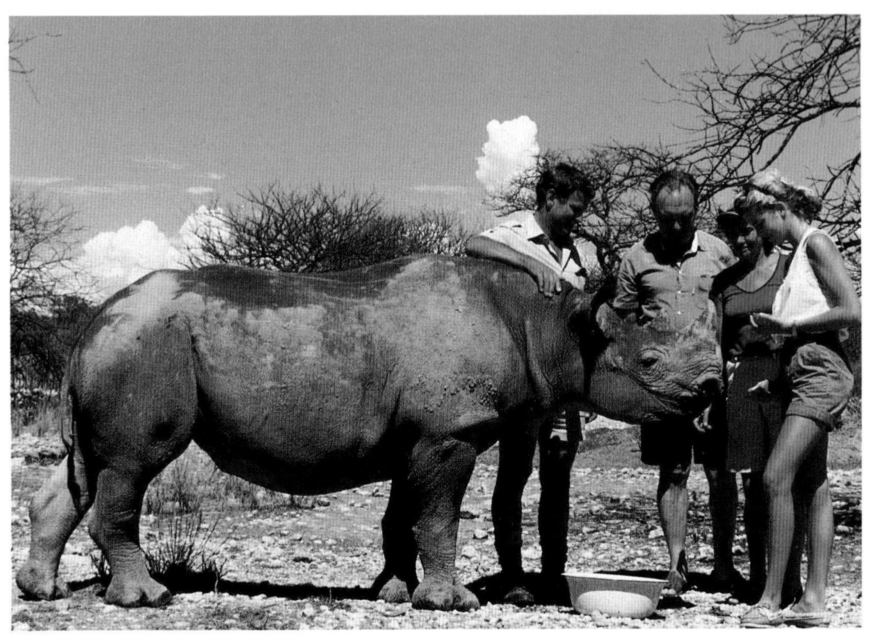

Additional drugs, derived from Haldol, are used to immobilize and capture dangerous animals for diagnostic testing, surgery, or transportation.

Haldol was R 1625, it was automatically referred to Searle in the late 1950's. Searle had the opportunity to develop and make the drug available to the U.S. market, but did not recognize the potential of Haldol.

In 1961 when Johnson & Johnson acquired Janssen Pharmaceutica, Searle had neither developed nor explicitly refused to develop Haldol, thus leaving it open for development by another company. The impasse was ended by J&J buying from Searle the United States rights to all Janssen compounds.

Johnson & Johnson made Haldol available to McNeil, the pharmaceutical company J&J had acquired prior to Janssen. While this opened an opportunity for McNeil to develop a major drug, McNeil management was opposed to Haldol. After four years McNeil had still not started clinical trials on the drug. As Dr. Janssen has remarked of that period, "The problem was convincing McNeil to do something."

There were two other obstacles that blocked Haldol's entry into the United States. One was the fact that American psychiatrists were, by the early 1960's, accustomed to using chlorpromazine, and other phenothiazine neuroleptics, whose performance was different from that of Haldol. Few psychiatrists were interested in this new drug. It was not that Haldol was inferior to the phenothiazines, but its speed of action and its effects were different from what American psychiatrists were accustomed to. In time, sufficient numbers of American psychiatrists were persuaded to try Haldol so that the clinical data needed for FDA approval was obtained. Subsequently, Haldol was used very extensively by American physicians, as it still is.

The second obstacle was the findings of the early American clinical trials. The results were negative and discouraging, with the initial report suggesting that Haldol was of little, if any, use. It reported serious side effects among patients who took it. A later, related report suggested that the different ethnic compositions of American and Belgian patients resulted in Haldol having very different effects in the two countries and that ten times as much Haldol was needed for American patients as for their Belgian counterparts to get the same results. The impact of these reports, of course, tended to discourage management at Searle and McNeil as well as other American physicians.

After almost 30 years, Haldol has been proved repeatedly to be one of the best — perhaps the best — of all known neuroleptics. Yet no one would have predicted this from these early American reports. It is a vivid warning to all concerned that early clinical reports about a compound must be treated with great circumspection. Results may even be reversed by later larger clinical trials conducted by more skillful physicians with perhaps more appropriate presuppositions than those who ran the early American trials on Haldol.

Another barrier which McNeil had to overcome before Haldol could be made available was the fact that regulations for drug approval had been changed. Before the thalidomide tragedy of the early 1960's, it was relatively easy to get a new drug approved, with only safety data required. But the Kefauver Amendments of 1962 to the Food, Drug and Cosmetics Act required much more extensive testing to show safety. They also imposed the unprecedented requirement that the effectiveness of each drug be demonstrated in detailed and lengthy clinical trials.

These changes caused difficulties and slowdowns for innovative pharmaceutical firms. The difficulties may have been worse for the McNeil executives who were trying to get Haldol approved. There was the problem of communicating with the Janssen people across the Atlantic Ocean and convincing them that evidence which had sufficed to get Haldol approved in France, West Germany, or Finland was not adequate for the United States.

The Janssen people and their McNeil colleagues had to learn what the FDA considered convincing evidence of effectiveness. Moreover, everybody involved in this regulatory activity was very well aware that in the aftermath of thalidomide, FDA personnel were much more likely to be commended by their superiors and the American public if they prevented a dangerous or ineffective drug from reaching people than if they approved a safe and effective drug.

The precipitous drop in the number of new pharmaceutical compounds approved annually in the United States in the years following passage of the Kefauver Amendments demonstrates vividly how difficult the new situation became for drug companies. The fact that Haldol was approved in the first few years after this enormous regulatory change shows what effective work was done by those involved, even though the sometimes impatient people in Beerse would have preferred that the approval come more quickly.

Haldol was a major American drug by the late 1960's. Yet it remained on patent until 1986. The reason involves an entanglement with Smith Kline & French, the company that introduced chlorpromazine in the United States. SK&F was researching many compounds that might have neuroleptic properties. This work was being done in the mid- and late-1950's when the Janssen researchers were finding their butyrophenone compounds.

Dr. Janssen had a friend, a European medicinal chemist, with whom he spoke frequently. He gave him a good deal of information about his own firm's research on neuroleptics. This friend was a consultant to SK&F and there has been speculation about whether he turned information about Janssen research over to his employers.

Whatever the facts, the United States Patent Office stopped its normal deliberations over the Haldol patent and announced what is called an "interference," an action the Patent Office takes when it is faced with applications from two or more sources for a patent on the same product. The Haldol application included compounds similar to Haldol, a protective patent device widely used when filing for patent protection. One of the compounds in the Janssen application was identical to one of the compounds in a patent application filed by SK&F. The Patent Office required an investigation to determine which applicant had discovered the compound first.

The patent dispute that ensued was relatively amicable. SK&F took a very reasonable position and the Patent Office finally ruled in favor of Janssen. When this ruling was made in 1969, the Haldol patent was granted. Seventeen years later, in 1986, Haldol's U.S. patent expired.

A Haldol derivative, Haldol Decanoate, R 13672, is now

available as a long-lasting drug whose chief appeal is that one injection provides the patient with protection for four weeks. The value of this form of Haldol for schizophrenics who are living in the community without daily medical supervision is quite clear, but that does not guarantee that patients who need the drug will report at four-week intervals to doctors who can give the needed injections. Haldol Decanoate is protected by a five-year patent extension in the United States under the 1984 Waxman-Hatch Amendments to the Food, Drug and Cosmetics Act.

Janssen chemists also synthesized an S_2 antagonist, R 3345, pipamperone, brand name Dipiperon. This neuroleptic was derived from haloperidol but its effects were distinctively different. Pipamperone improves sleep, a property not possessed by Haldol. At higher doses, it is antiautistic, disinhibiting and resocializing, all effects useful in treating chronic psychoses. It also has the virtue of being unlikely to produce extrapyramidal symptoms. Additional research produced other neuroleptics such as bromperidol, R 11333, made available under the trade name Impromen, along with its long-acting form, bromperidol decanoate, R 46541, sold under the brand name Impromen Decanoate.

The 1980's have witnessed a new wave of neuroleptics that differ dramatically from those created from the Haldol model. One of the most brilliant stars in this new Janssen galaxy is risperidone, R 64766. How it came to be is a classic example of how Janssen research works. Janssen explorers integrated the general knowledge produced by the rapid advance of science with the lessons learned from Janssen accomplishments in the past. Researchers knew that improved drugs against psychosis might be obtained by finding an appropriate S_2 antagonist, or by finding drugs which were simultaneously D_2 and S_2 antagonists.

In 1981, these insights led Janssen chemists to synthesize setoperone, R 52245. This was a much more potent S_2 antagonist than pipamperone had been, and it was also a moderate dopamine antagonist. At the extreme left of setoperone we have a thiazole and a pyrimidine ring, sharing a common nitrogen atom. But even setoperone retained the core of the haloperidol structure, the piperidine ring preceded by a CH_2 fragment, presumably the part of the molecule producing some degree of dopamine antagonism. This combination of a serotonin and a dopamine antagonist produced improvements in chronic schizophrenic patients, mainly in emotional withdrawal, tension, depressed mood, and blunted feelings. Setoperone also produced much less extrapyramidal symptomatology than other neuroleptic therapies.

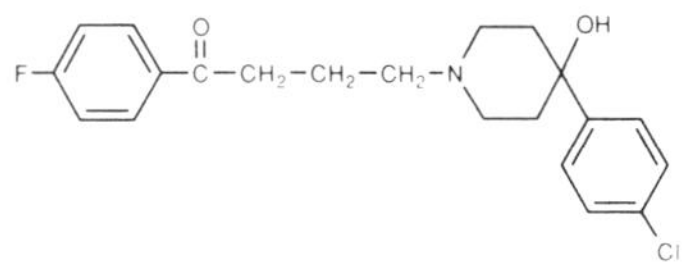

HALOPERIDOL

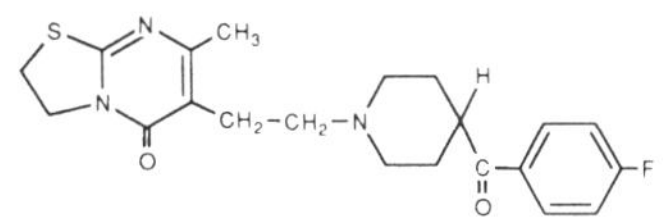

SETOPERONE

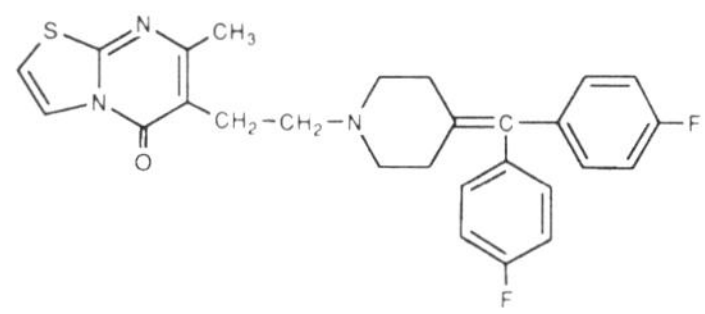

RITANSERIN

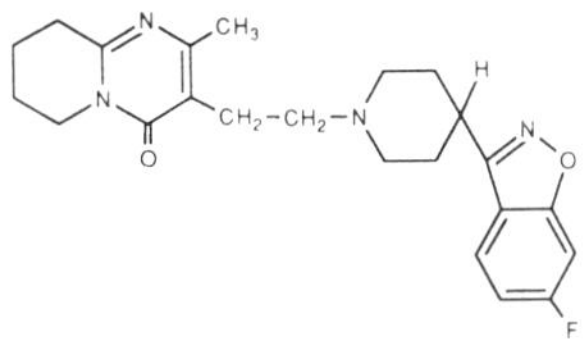

RISPERIDONE

Nevertheless, setoperone had serious deficiencies. Its weak dopamine antagonism made it inferior to haloperidol in those respects in which the latter neuroleptic was most effective. Also setoperone's bioavailability of less than one percent made it difficult to work with. So Janssen researchers turned to a pure S_2 antagonist R 55667, ritanserin, which had been synthesized in 1982.

Ritanserin is identical with setoperone on the left-hand side. The changes come on the right-hand side beyond the piperidine ring where the carbonyl (C=O) combination and the single hydrogen atom directly attached to the piperidine in setoperone have been dropped. Instead the piperidine is followed by a double-bonded carbon atom which in turn connects with two benzene rings, each of which is linked to a fluorine atom.

Ritanserin had earlier been shown to have extraordinary effects on human sleep, specifically increasing the duration of slow-wave sleep. This deep sleep may be doubled by ritanserin, and it is obviously very important in the restorative powers of sleep. This phase of sleep was known to be deeply disturbed in schizophrenic patients. For these reasons it was decided that ritanserin would be tried in a double-blind clinical trial in schizophrenic patients. The normal neuroleptic therapy for these patients was continued, but one group had ritanserin added while the second had a placebo added to the usual therapy.

The results of this double-blind study were striking. It became clear in comparison with the placebo that ritanserin improved mainly the negative and affective symptoms such as anxiety, depression, lack of energy and activity. Moreover, extrapyramidal symptoms declined significantly in the patients who received ritanserin, while there was also a significant reduction of tremor, an effect similar to that reported in a clinical trial of ritanserin on patients with Parkinson's disease.

Thought was given to making ritanserin available as a supplemental therapy for schizophrenia, one capable of producing improved results if administered with haloperidol or others of the classical dopamine antagonists. But against this was the obvious utility and convenience of an antipsychotic therapy consisting of one drug. Ideally, such a drug would combine the positive effects of haloperidol-like drugs and the useful effects of ritanserin.

The desired drug turned out to be R 64766, risperidone, which was synthesized in 1984. The left-hand side of risperidone had one major change from the structural formulas of setoperone and ritanserin. Instead of the extreme left-hand ring being a thiazole ring, risperidone has a piperidine ring there, one that shares a nitrogen atom with the adjoining pyrimidine ring. On the right-hand side of risperidone, just beyond the piperidine ring, there is now an upper hydrogen atom just as there is in setoperone. In the lower part at the extreme right of risperidone are two rings joined together.

The upper is an isoxazole ring with a nitrogen and an oxygen atom at two adjoining vertices, while beneath that is a benzene ring with a fluorine atom attached.

Risperidone has been tested on psychotic patients with florid delusions and great difficulty in making normal human contact. It has shown that it has effective antidelusional action, significantly improving patients' moods and ability to make contacts with others. In short, as a drug which is both an S_2 and a D_2 antagonist, risperidone apparently is able to combat what psychiatrists call both the positive and negative defects of schizophrenia. It appears to do this with much less likelihood of extrapyramidal symptoms than exists in the classic dopamine antagonists of the chlorpromazine and haloperidol generation of antipsychotic drugs.

Risperidone is still only in mid-passage in the long gauntlet of clinical trials and other tests that a new therapy must surmount. It could still be abandoned because of some new development. But even if that happens, it is likely that Janssen researchers have other compounds available with similar remarkable powers.

The quest which began in the mid-1950's continues. That is the nature of research. It is the way of life for Paul Janssen and his team of researchers. Better medicines will always be needed. Often they are found with one eye reviewing the past and the other searching for new paths to future discoveries.

Chapter 6

IN THE CONQUEST OF PAIN

The conquest of pain has always been a major objective of human beings, going back long before the birth of modern medicine and medical science. Throughout history, folk remedies have claimed to be helpful for this purpose. Opium's utility for easing pain during surgery was apparently realized and used more than 2000 years ago, although not on a scientific basis. For centuries alcohol has been known to relieve pain. It was frequently used throughout the nineteenth century during amputation procedures.

But the routine control of pain, in both daily life and in surgery, which we take for granted, has only been available in the last century or so. George Washington, Napoleon Bonaparte, Abraham Lincoln, and Louis Pasteur had no tablet readily available which would relieve even the most insistent headache. And in past centuries it was not infrequent that a person needing an amputation or other serious surgery was simply bound hand and foot and the surgery proceeded without anesthesia.

Over the past 36 years, Dr. Paul Janssen and his collaborators have written a major chapter in the history of coping with pain, especially surgical pain. In over 50 countries, one or more of the compounds discovered at Beerse are used routinely for the relief of moderate to severe pain. Wherever modern surgery is performed, anesthesia with a Janssen product is a frequent daily reality.

In November 1984, when William J. Schroeder received his artificial heart at the Humana Hospital in Louisville, Kentucky, it was a Janssen anesthetic, Sufenta (sufentanil), R 33800, which was employed. Mr. Schroeder lived longer than any other person who has received that device. Murray Hayden, the next person to receive an artificial heart, also had his operation under Sufenta anesthesia.

Dr. P. Shanahan, the anesthesiologist at both operations, said, "The surgical intervention on W.J. Schroeder was extremely difficult because a lot of scar tissue had already developed as the result of an earlier bypass operation. This is why the operation was scheduled to last six-and-one-half hours, which is two hours longer than the first artificial heart patient, Dr. Barney Clark. Sufenta was used throughout the entire period and was subsequently administered in a low dose as a sedative for 36 hours after the operation. I chose Sufenta because it has a minimal influence on the hemodynamics. I don't think Schroeder could have survived this intervention without the progress which is heralded by the new anesthetic." Sufentanil was still considered an experimental drug by the FDA when it was used in the surgery. It did not receive formal clearance in the United States until two years later.

Narcotic analgesics and anesthetics are the pain killers with which the Janssen name is associated. The Janssen anesthetic agents are infused intravenously, rather than inhaled like ether, nitrous oxide, and chloroform, which opened the era of anesthesia in the mid-nineteenth century. These inhalant agents revolutionized surgery in the nineteenth century by permitting the surgeon to take his time since the patient was asleep and in no distress. They also vastly increased the number and variety of operations which could be performed safely.

But for all their great utility, these original inhalant anesthetic agents had disadvantages which induced surgeons and anesthesiologists to keep looking for better compounds. Ether, for example, is relatively safe and potent and has superior muscle relaxant properties. But it is flammable, irritating to the upper airway and has an unpleasant odor. Today it has been largely replaced by other inhalant and intravenous anesthetics that are free from these disadvantages.

Nitrous oxide, the most widely used inhalant anesthetic, is a weak anesthetic. When it is used, a barbiturate is first employed to produce hypnosis, and later anesthesia is maintained with the help of another inhalant or a narcotic analgesic. Chloroform has a very narrow safety margin between an effective dose and a lethal dose, a very serious drawback to its frequent use.

Morphine, the active analgesic ingredient in opium, was isolated in 1806, but its use in medicine required the invention of the syringe and the hollow needle, devices which did not become available until after 1850. By about 1870, physicians began studying morphine for premedication before an operation. They also began using subcutaneous doses for minor surgery. Around 1900, morphine and scopolamine began to be used for surgical anesthesia, but several patients died and this use was abandoned.

The first half of this century saw the introduction of several morphine derivatives as well as the first entirely synthetic opiate, a compound known as meperidine or pethidine. But narcotic anesthesia still was not widely employed because it always held the threat of respiratory depression — that the patient might stop breathing and die. Dr. Janssen was interested in narcotic analgesia as early as 1953 when his professional research work began. That research resulted in a triumph, the compound known as Palfium (dextromoramide) or R 874, which was synthesized in 1956. A quarter of a century later in 1981, Dr. Janssen wrote of that discovery, "Today, dextromoramide is still available in more than 50 countries for the treatment of severe pain. It is used both parenterally and orally. For us, dextromoramide has become a compound of merely historical significance."

Dextromoramide is related to methadone, which is perhaps a clue to the research path that resulted in its discovery. Two things about this compound are worth noting.

First, the main axis of the compound begins with two benzene rings which are separated horizontally by three carbon atoms from the nitrogen atom of the morpholine six-membered ring — a piperidine ring with the fourth carbon atom replaced by an oxygen atom. For some years, the Janssen researchers believed that this arrangement was a prerequisite for a successful narcotic analgesic, and they did indeed find several other analgesics with this same structural spine.

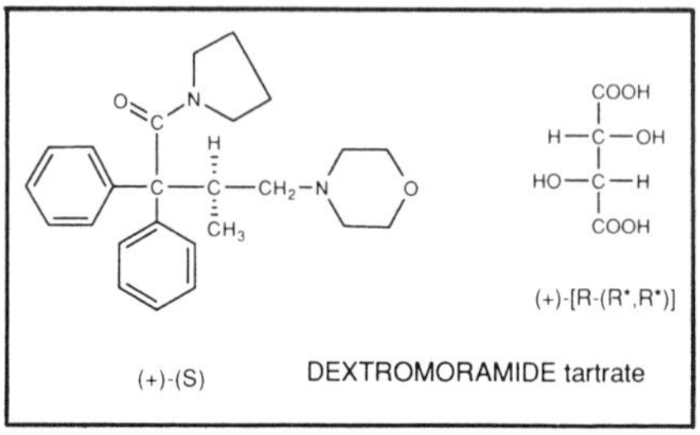

(+)-[R-(R*,R*)]

(+)-(S) DEXTROMORAMIDE tartrate

Second, beginning with dextromoramide, Dr. Janssen was using as a measure of analgesic power the tail withdrawal test. Pain is a subjective phenomenon to which human beings can testify. But animals can't talk and so tests of pain and of diminution of pain have to be based on their objective responses. In the tail withdrawal test in rats, the objective behavior which is measured is the speed with which a rat removes its tail from hot water, maintained at a constant temperature of 55 degrees Centigrade, 131 degrees Fahrenheit. Normal unmedicated rats, used as controls, will remove their tails within 3 to 5 seconds after immersion.

In rats treated with opiate analgesics, the tail removal may be delayed or completely blocked. The degree to which treated rats delay tail removal is a measure of how much pain relief the medication has given them. Moreover, by measuring the tail withdrawal time at different periods after treatment, it is possible to evaluate the onset of the analgesic effect, the time of peak effect, and the total duration of analgesia.

Rats injected subcutaneously with dextromoramide showed fast onset of analgesia, a peak effect at one-half hour after injection and a duration of pain relief for about as long as was secured with methadone and meperidine. Rats injected with a dose of dextromoramide equal to 0.2 milligram per kilogram of the animal's weight took between six and ten seconds to remove their tails from the hot water, suggesting some weak analgesic effect.

Those injected with a dose almost twice as great, 0.37 mg per kg of animal body weight, took longer than 10 seconds to remove their tails. This suggested they had analgesia sufficient for surgery. By this test it was possible to show that dextromoramide was about 10 times more potent than methadone, 25 times more potent than morphine, and 50 times more potent than meperidine.

Shortly after he had discovered dextromoramide, Dr. Janssen began using meperidine with its piperidine ring structure as the model analgesic, looking for variations of other, more effective analgesics and anesthetics. Morphine, of course, is the original narcotic analgesic, but it has a very complicated structure. That great complexity of structure explains why morphine has so many effects on living organisms. But the chemist looking for new compounds prefers a simpler structure as a starting point, and meperidine has a much simpler structure than morphine. Dextromoramide is the only Janssen analgesic compound which does not contain a piperidine ring: instead it has a morpholine ring.

Three other significant analgesics have been discovered and made available by Janssen Pharmaceutica. In 1957, phenoperidine, R 1406, was synthesized; in 1960, piritramide, R 3365, and in 1961, bezitramide, R 4845. All three have piperidine rings and horizontal axes on which a benzene ring at the extreme left is separated by three carbon atoms from the nitrogen atom which is part of the piperidine ring.

Phenoperidine is a potent, fast, and short-acting morphine-like analgesic that has been and is still used in anesthesia. Piritramide is roughly as potent as morphine, has a similar duration of action and a somewhat faster onset. It has been used for postoperative pain relief and its big advantage over other morphine-like analgesics is the infrequency of nausea and vomiting as side effects.

Bezitramide is a highly potent oral analgesic with a slow onset of action, a long duration of about 12 hours, and an insolubility believed to diminish its potential for abuse. It is particularly useful in terminal cancer patients.

But it is in the related field of anesthesia that Janssen

Pharmaceutica has really made its major pain-relief impact on world medicine. The formal pioneers in that specialty were two Belgian anesthesiologists, Drs. J. De Castro and R. Mundeleer, who worked at the University of Brussels in the late 1950s. At a conference in 1959 they proposed the use of neuroleptanalgesia (NLA) for intravenous anesthesia, or the use of only two drugs, a neuroleptic and a strong narcotic, for anesthesia purposes in major surgery. Initially, they used haloperidol and phenoperidine, but shortly thereafter they switched to two other Janssen drugs, the neuroleptic Inapsine (droperidol), or R 4749, and the narcotic Sublimaze (fentanyl), R 4263.

The rationale was that surgery produces stress and pain, and anesthesia can guard against both by using a combination of a neuroleptic and an analgesic. Additionally, the neuroleptic droperidol produces tranquilization and sedation while acting to prevent the vomiting often produced by morphine and morphine-like analgesics. Fentanyl contributes sedation and analgesia, but produces depressed respiration which can be solved by a mechanical ventilator to regulate breathing.

NLA did not fully guarantee against the patient retaining some consciousness during the surgery and having memories of it. But this could be solved by administering either nitrous oxide or a hypnotic drug such as one of the benzodiazepines.

An American professor of anesthesiology advised Dr. Janssen that droperidol and fentanyl should be together in a fixed combination, one part fentanyl and 50 parts droperidol. This resulted in a drug made available under the brand name, Innovar. This was done to prevent the abuse of fentanyl, a narcotic, outside the field of anesthesia. Subsequently Janssen has successfully marketed fentanyl alone.

Many years later the same policy was followed with two other major Janssen anesthesia products, Sufenta (sufentanil), or R 33800, a potent narcotic analgesic, and Alfenta (alfentanil), or R 39209, the shortest-acting narcotic analgesic known. Alfentanil offers great advantages for surgical procedures of brief duration. Mechanical ventilation may still be necessary with alfentanil but recovery is so fast that the patient can go home in a few hours.

It is notable that over the past three decades regulatory approval time has lengthened appreciably for anesthetic agents as well as other drugs in general. Fentanyl was first synthesized in 1960 and was being used only three years later. Sufentanil, first synthesized in 1974, did not become available until five years later. Finally, alfentanil, first synthesized in 1976, was approved seven years later.

In the 1960s, cardiac surgeons and anesthesiologists began to experiment with anesthesia consisting only of very high doses of morphine. To the surprise of many anesthesiologists, high-dose morphine anesthesia turned out to be usable and to have some key advantages. But it had enough drawbacks so that anesthesiologists turned their attention to replacing the morphine with high doses of fentanyl, a substitution that many anesthesiologists found advantageous.

Later, when sufentanil became available, it proved suitable for use as an anesthetic as a single agent, particularly in high risk and stressful procedures, such as open heart surgery. Since sufentanil is much more potent than fentanyl, the amount required for anesthesia is less than the comparable amounts of fentanyl and morphine.

Fentanyl, alone or in combination with droperidol, has been and is being used widely throughout the world by many anesthesiologists. The NLA combination has played a historic role in the world development of anesthesiological practice. Sufentanil and alfentanil are of much more recent vintage and have only in recent years begun to come into the mainstream of anesthesia practice.

In the United States, sufentanil was not approved until 1985 and alfentanil until 1987. Anesthesiologists are constantly looking for better anesthetic agents since no one drug or combination of drugs meets all needs. However, Harvard anesthesia Professor Edward Lowenstein told a 1983 symposium at the Cleveland Clinic, "I believe narcotic anesthesia will continue to thrive." There is no obvious reason to challenge his confidence.

Fentanyl, sufentanil, and alfentanil differ from the analgesics discussed above in that they all have a phenylanilino group very close to the piperidine ring. The phenylanilino group consists of the phenyl or benzene ring with the nitrogen atom just above it, all of which are immediately to the lower right of the piperidine ring.

Only fentanyl has a benzene ring at its extreme left. The five-sided ring at the extreme left of sufentanil is an isosteric 2-thienyl moiety, a pentagon with a sulfur atom at one vertex as well as carbon atoms at the other four vertices. The 2-thienyl moiety and the phenyl or benzene ring are isosteric because they both have similar chemical properties, though they are composed of different kinds and numbers of atoms. Finally, alfentanil has a very novel structure on its left side, the tetrazolinone ring, a pentagon containing an oxygen atom and four nitrogen atoms.

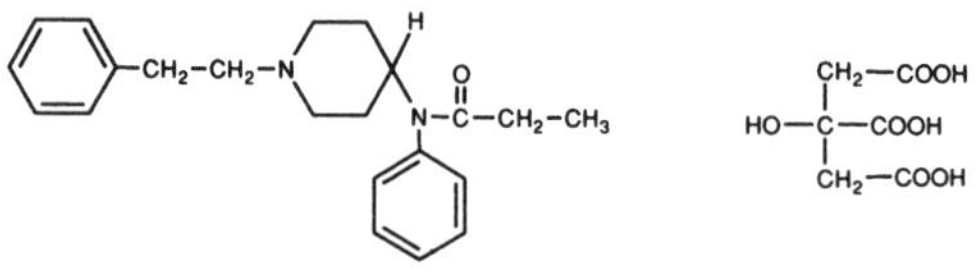

FENTANYL citrate

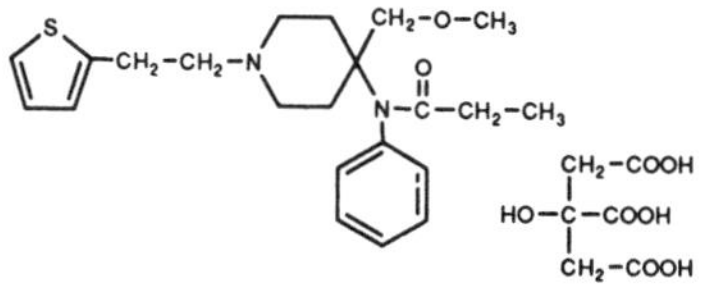

SUFENTANIL citrate

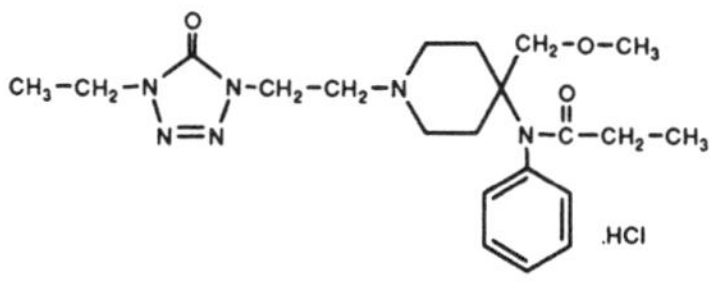

ALFENTANIL hydrochloride

Dr. Wim Van Bever has explained the genesis of the idea. "We already knew that the phenyl group in the side chain could be replaced isosterically by another aromatic group, for instance by 2-thienyl (as for sufentanil). Since we wanted a short-acting compound, I suggested replacing the rather stable phenyl group by a metabolically vulnerable quasi-aromatic tetrazolone moiety, which indeed turned out to give rise to very short-acting compounds."

How were these different analgesic and anesthetic agents

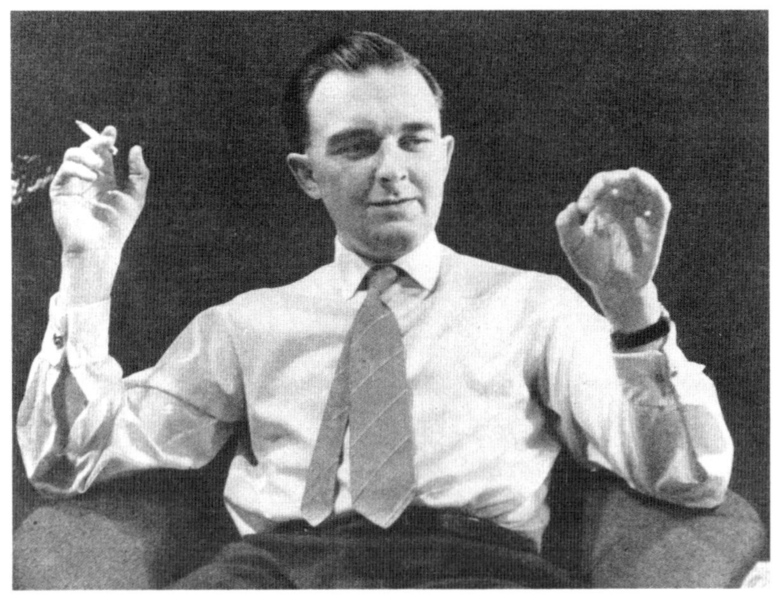

News of a new drug more powerful than morphine came to international attention in 1955. A reporter, covering a Paris medical conference, learned of Paul Janssen's conquest of pain. The press wanted to know about the new medicine, Palfium, and about the young scientist.

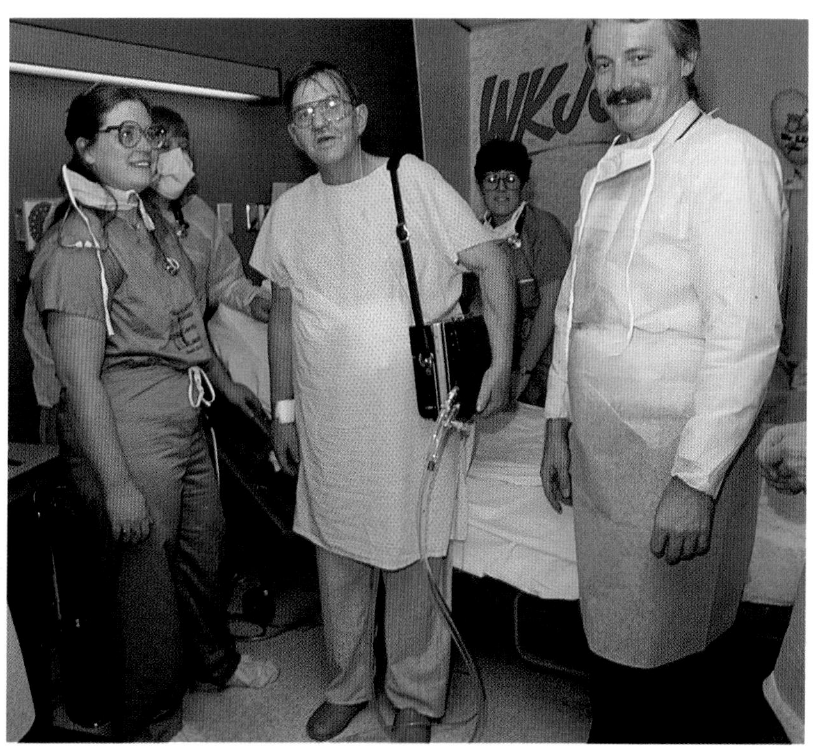

William Schroeder's artifical heart ushered in a new era in medical breakthroughs. The six-and-a-half hour surgical procedure was performed with a Janssen anesthestic, Sufenta. "I don't think Schroeder could have survived this intervention without the progress which is heralded by the new anesthetics," commented the anesthesiologist.

discovered? The basic process is one we have discussed before, taking a starting compound and modifying it in many ways, meanwhile studying the changing effects of each modification carefully. Those effects which appear to improve the molecule in terms of desired results are built upon further in a search that can encompass hundreds or even thousands of new compounds prepared and tested in the hunt for the desired end product.

All these compounds have a common skeleton including such units as the piperidine ring and the phenylanilino group very nearby. As new compounds based on this skeleton were synthesized and tested, the findings were recorded in computers and studied to see what patterns emerged that might guide further exploration. A hint of the huge amount of work that goes into these efforts can be seen in the scholarly studies Dr. Janssen and his collaborators have published to systematize and make available their anesthesia findings and those of others.

In April 1962, Dr. Janssen published an article in the *British Journal of Anesthesia*, "A Review of the Chemical Features Associated with Strong Morphine-Like Activity." He began by asserting, "It appears safe to presume that all potent narcotics exert their effects by a common mechanism of action. If this is true, then it appears reasonable to look for chemical features that are associated with morphine-like activity, particularly among narcotics producing their effects at low-dose levels. There might indeed exist something like a common specific receptor area, somewhere in the brain, possibly in the thalamic area, to which a narcotic molecule must be able to fit before it can act. No one has ever demonstrated this hypothetical area, of course, and there is no serious reason to believe that anyone will be able to do so in the near future. We might, therefore, try to approach the problem from the opposite angle and ascertain to what extent molecules with powerful narcotic properties look alike chemically."

He discussed different types of compounds with morphine-like analgesia and summarized his findings in a three-dimensional model representing the common chemical features associated with morphine-like activity at low-dose levels. He concluded by stating, "Because these molecules look alike chemically, it appears reasonable to assume that there might be something like a common receptor for morphine-like drugs."

A decade after this article, Drs. Solomon Snyder and Candace Pert of Johns Hopkins University demonstrated that they had found morphine receptors in the brain. In fact, it was soon found that the brain naturally contains morphine-like analgesic compounds of its own manufacture. As Dr. Janssen had surmised in 1962, the thalamus has numerous opiate receptors.

By 1968, Janssen researchers knew even more about compounds that might provide morphine-like analgesia. This formidable array of data was published in an article written by Dr. Janssen and Cyriel A.M. Van der Eycken, titled, "The Chemical Anatomy of Potent Morphine-Like Analgesics." It summed up the findings of research on hundreds of compounds whose properties as morphine-like analgesics had been studied in various species. It concluded with generalizations as to which properties of different types of compounds seemed to favor high analgesic power. The article became a basic source of ideas for further analgesia and anesthesia research, not only for Janssen researchers but for their competitors and in many universities engaged in pharmacological research.

The brain has at least four receptors for opiates. These have been and are still being studied assiduously by scientists in many countries. Two Janssen compounds are used widely for studying these brain receptors, sufentanil and lofentanil, R 34995. Lofentanil is a highly potent and very long-acting narcotic analgesic. To study brain opiate receptors, both compounds are made radioactive by the incorporation of tritium, a radioactive form of hydrogen. Using these compounds, the distribution of opiate receptors in the brain can be charted because, on administering these compounds intravenously, the distribution of radioactivity in the brain becomes proportional to the number of opiate receptors in different parts of that organ.

A paper detailing the many Janssen compounds now used to investigate different receptors in the human organism was the lead article in the May-August 1986 issue of *Drug Development Research*, a festschrift or commemorative publication, prepared by Dr. Janssen's research associates to mark his 60th birthday and 33 years of drug development research.

Twenty years passed between the synthesis of the first Janssen narcotic analgesic, dextromoramide, and the synthesis of alfentanil. These were two decades of intensive and highly fruitful research into all aspects of the control of pain. This research yielded drugs for clinical analgesia and anesthesia as well as a rich harvest of basic scientific information about pain perception in living organisms and the compounds and receptors involved in this perception and its modification.

Chapter 7

PIONEERS AGAINST PARASITIC DISEASE

When the Belgian Congo gained its independence and became the nation of Zaire in 1960, the consequences of such a change were of enormous importance to many countries and industries. A completely unexpected result was that Janssen Pharmaceutica became a world pioneer and leader in finding and producing medicines against parasitic diseases. These ailments afflict a large portion of the human race as well as vast numbers of domestic animals such as pigs, sheep, cattle, chickens, horses, and dogs.

These diseases, caused mainly by worms, protozoa, and fungi, exact enormous tolls each year in deaths and suffering. Most of the human victims are in the developing nations of Africa, Asia, and Latin America. But there are also significant numbers in the poorer areas of the industrialized world. Innumerable domestic animals in all parts of the world suffer and sometimes die from these diseases.

In 1960, the long arm of coincidence provided the link between the political events in the Congo and Janssen research. It actually began in the summer of 1926 in the Belgian town of Turnhout where two boys, Robert Marsboom and Paul Janssen, were born. The Marsboom and Janssen families lived within 500 yards of each other and came from the same socioeconomic group. The head of the Janssen family was one of the town's few physicians, while the head of the Marsboom family was the town's top local government administrator.

Robert and Paul got to know each other when they were

about five years old. They grew up together, going to the same school, often in the same class, and frequently playing soccer together. When it was time to go to the university, they both went to the University of Ghent; Paul to become a physician and Robert to become a veterinary surgeon.

After graduation, their paths diverged. After receiving his veterinary degree, Dr. Marsboom received a degree in tropical medicine from the Institute of Tropical Medicine in Antwerp. He went to the Belgian Congo as a government agent assigned to help prevent disease in the large domestic animal population of the area. The Belgian government was very anxious to recruit the best possible talent for the Congo. It provided such incentives as high salaries and long home leaves with all expenses paid. These jobs appealed to adventurous young Belgians who wanted to travel outside their country to the challenges of tropical Central Africa.

Dr. Marsboom broadened his knowledge about the frequent interrelationships between human and animal diseases. He traveled widely because the diseases were often spread by insects, particularly the tsetse fly (sleeping sickness) and the anopheles mosquito (malaria). These problems were common in both the Congo and in the British colonies which are now the nations of Kenya, Uganda, and Tanzania. Dr. Marsboom had accumulated ten years of rich practical experience in Central Africa when the Belgian government announced the Congo's independence. That news forced him and other Belgians working in the Congo to ponder their futures.

Dr. Marsboom must have been one of the first Belgians to decide in 1960 to go back home and start a new career. Having made that decision, he thought of his old friend Dr. Paul Janssen who, he believed, was working hard with patients in Turnhout. Dr. Marsboom wrote to Janssen and received a prompt reply requesting that he come join Janssen Pharmaceutica as soon as possible. On October 15, 1960, Dr. Robert Marsboom arrived at the Janssen laboratories in Beerse bringing his personal microscope with him, one of a very small number of microscopes on the premises.

Dr. Marsboom's skills were needed immediately in the breeding chambers for laboratory animals, almost all of which were mice and rats. The animals were not mating and therefore not reproducing. Using his microscope, Dr. Marsboom examined several of the animals and in five minutes had the problem solved. The decreased libido was caused by a severe infestation of mites among the laboratory animals.

His African experience had showed him the solution. He recommended that the animals be submerged briefly in a tank containing an appropriate solution which would cleanse them of their mites, thus ending the itching and restoring the animals' normal interest in procreation. His advice was followed and the breeding crisis was soon over.

The incident demonstrated how little Dr. Janssen and his group of 150 people knew about animal medicine. But Dr. Marsboom's arrival did more than give the Janssen enterprise its own expert veterinarian. Additionally, Dr. Marsboom began to educate his old friend and new colleagues in the many areas of medicine arising from parasitic infections in human beings and animals — medical topics of which the scientists in Beerse knew very little.

Dr. Marsboom encouraged his colleagues to take a fresh look at existing Janssen compounds. Perhaps some could be used in animal medicine. He pointed out that Janssen had some products that could be useful for veterinarians and livestock breeders. A Dr. Marcel Rogiers was particularily interested in the problems surrounding the behavior of pigs. Pigs are aggressive animals and in general susceptible to stress. When pigs from different origins are brought together, many problems can arise, such as fighting and injury. Weight loss and even deaths can occur.

Azaperone, R 1929, a neuroleptic, was developed as a tranquilizer for animals. Azaperone became a management tool for pig breeders, allowing them to mix piglets in fattening pens and to transport them to market with no fighting or weight loss. Dr. Rogiers left his practice in 1971 to join Janssen, and today is vice president for the Animal Health Division.

Once the Janssen researchers learned of the importance of parasitic diseases on the world scene, they sought to find new compounds that might attack these diseases in man and animals. But Dr. Janssen would need additional personnel with the interest, training, and experience for such research. Once Dr. Marsboom had resumed his warm friendship and mutual trust with Dr. Janssen, he recruited other experts in veterinary medicine who wanted to leave the Congo. Over the next few years, several dozen of the best of the Flemish specialists from the Belgian Congo joined Janssen Pharmaceutica. These newcomers greatly expanded and diversified the skills, capabilities, and directions of Janssen research.

One of the most important recruits was Dr. Denis Thienpont, a veterinarian who had gone to the Congo in 1945. Widely respected by his colleagues, Dr. Thienpont had been director of the School for Veterinary Medicine in Butare (Ruanda) for ten years. He had had the opportunity to expand his original training and knowledge from the Congo experience and from the growing volume of new knowledge arising in veterinary medicine. This knowledge was also often complementary and directly related to the rapidly increasing knowledge of human medicine and diseases.

In 1962 when Dr. Marsboom recruited Dr. Thienpont to join the Janssen research team, he brought one of the Western world's outstanding experts in parasitic and fungal diseases to Beerse. Dr. Janssen, following his basic policy of building research around the interests and talents of his associates, immediately set up a Division of Worm and Fungal Diseases under Dr. Thienpont, who in effect received a charter to begin an energetic research program on these diseases.

Dr. Janssen referred to Dr. Thienpont as "my good friend, long-time collaborator and superb teacher in parasitology, mycology and protozoology." After the latter's retirement in 1982 the Janssen Research Foundation established a triennial Denis Thienpont Prize for Parasitology and Mycology, an award of $25,000 to individuals who have made important contributions to "fundamental or clinical knowledge in the field of parasitology or mycology." It is awarded under the auspices of the two branches (French and Flemish) of the Royal Academy of Medicine of Belgium.

A third key figure in the enormous progress against para-

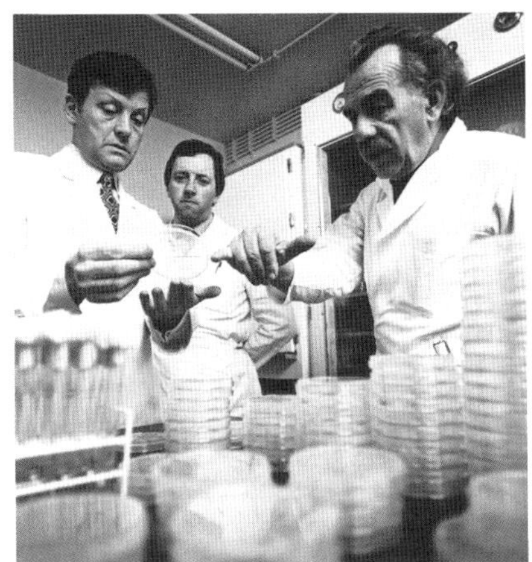

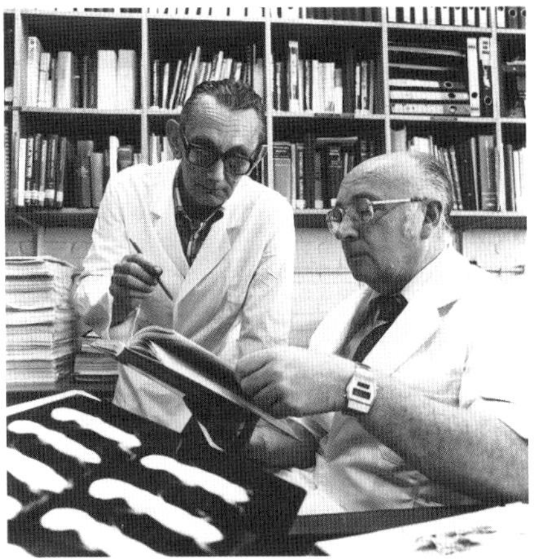

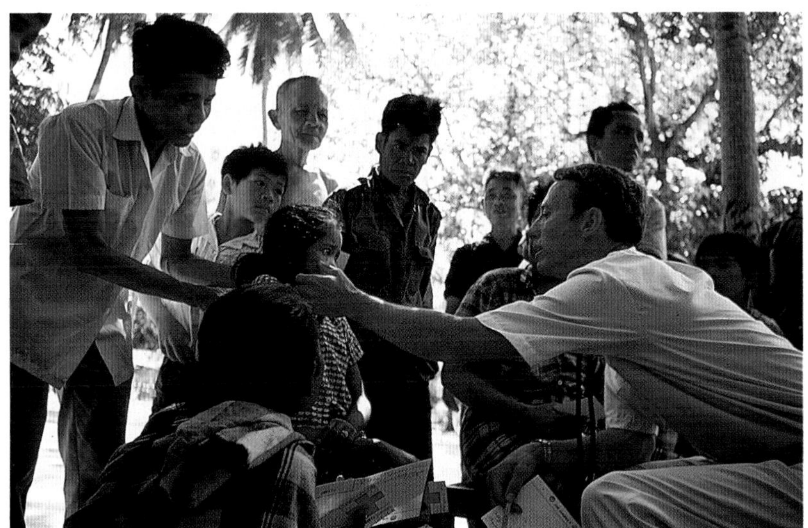

Dr. Denis Thienpont (foreground upper left) and Dr. Robert Marsboom (seated upper right), pioneers in the war against parasites, brought their years of field experience in the Congo to the Janssen research team. Their discoveries helped millions of people, especially in Third World countries.

THE NEW YORK TIMES, TUESDAY, OCTOBER 3, 1989

New Drug Treatment For Colon Cancer

BETHESDA, Md., Oct. 2 (AP) — A drug used to deworm farm animals combined with a common cancer drug has been found to save the lives of patients with an advanced type of colon cancer, the National Cancer Institute announced today.

The institute's director, Dr. Samuel Broder, said a national study involving about 1,300 patients with stage 3 colon cancer (on a four-stage scale) showed increased survival rates for those treated with a drug called levamisole in combination with 5-fluorouracil, a cancer drug now in common use.

The study was directed by Dr. Charles G. Moertel of the Mayo Clinic.

At a news conference today, Dr. Moertel said that the study showed 49 percent of the stage 3 colon cancer patients were alive five years after therapy with the drug combination, as against only 37 percent of such patients who received no drugs. Both of the patient groups being compared had been treated with surgery, wh... revealed that the colon... spread to...

cancer. The combination drug therapy is started three to five weeks after surgery and is continued for about a year.

Levamisole is used by veterinarians to clear worms from the intestines of barnyard animals. It is not now approved by the Food and Drug Administration for any human use in the United States. But the drug is

Advanced cases are found to benefit from a combination therapy.

commonly used in Europe... worm infestation i... has been wide... treatmen... Dr...

THE WALL STREET JOURNAL TUESDAY, JULY 18, 1989

A 'Miracle' Drug That Languished Among the Worms

By HARRY SCHWARTZ

The newest "miracle" cancer drug is levamisole. The Food and Drug Administration is permitting its distribution free of charge for use, together with another anti-cancer drug, 5-fluorouracil (5-FU), by individuals who have undergone surgery for colon cancer. Doctors involved in clinical tests with levamisole have expressed extraordinary enthusiasm for its potential in prolonging survival among these patients.

Lost in the public hurrahs for the new-found drug are some fundamental facts that ought to cause serious reflection among those in charge of new-drug approval in this country. Levamisole was first discovered more than a generation ago, in 1966, and its potential against cancer and other diseases was known by the early and mid-1970s. Yet it is only now, in 1989, that levamisole is entering the oncologist's arsenal.

Levamisole was discovered by the Belgian pharmacologist and chemist Paul Janssen and his team at Janssen Pharmaceutica, a firm—now a subsidiary of Johnson & Johnson—headquartered in the village of Beerse, near Antwerp. Since it began work in 1953, the Janssen team has discovered more than 70 drugs that are now in use or are in development—... larger number of drugs th...

THE WASHINGTON POST TUESDAY, OCTOBER 3, 1989

New Therapy Could Cut Colon Cancer Deaths

Drugs Would Be Used Along With Surgery

By Sandy Rovner
Washington Post Staff Writer

The death rate from advanced colon cancer, now the second leading cancer killer, could be reduced by one-third through the use of a newly developed combination of drugs, National Cancer Institute (NCI) officials announced yesterday.

The new treatment, which combines a veterinary de-worming agent with a standard anticancer drug and which was tested on 1,700 patients over the last eight years, is the first form of chemotherapy to be found effective against colon cancer. Even with surgery, the only treatment until now, nearly two-thirds of the patients died within five years. Now, with surgery plus drugs, that rate is expected to fall to about one-half.

Although the drug combination has not been approved by the Food and Drug Administration, the cancer officials said letters have gone out to 35,000 cancer doctors, alerting them to the treatment's effectiveness and its availability directly from NCI. The drugs are to be used only after surgery has removed the obvious tumors.

Tuesday, Oct. 3, 1989 The Philadelphia Inquirer

Colon cancer treatment could save thousands

By Jim Detjen
Inquirer Staff Writer

More than 3,000 lives could be saved each year if a new form of chemotherapy for colon cancer patients is used, researchers at the University of Pennsylvania and the National Cancer Institute said yesterday.

In two studies involving 1,704 cancer patients, including about 100 from the Philadelphia area, researchers found that death rates could be reduced 10 percent to 15 percent if two drugs were given after surgery.

The National Cancer Institute sent out a special announcement to 36,000 physicians and cancer researchers urging them to adopt the new treatment, if possible. Until yesterday, no drugs were recommended after surgery.

The new form of chemotherapy is a "significant advance" in the fight against colon cancer, the nation's second-leading cause of cancer deaths, said Daniel Haller, an associate professor at the University of Pennsylvania Cancer Center.

Michael Friedman, an associate director at NCI, called the new treatment an "important breakthrough" because of the large number of people it could help. This year, an estimated 53,500 Americans will die of colon cancer, second only to lung cancer, which will kill an estimated 142,000 people.

But Haller, who participated in the research, cautioned that the drugs had been found to be effective only when used on patients who had undergone surgery for colon cancer and who had cancer that had spread to adjacent lymph nodes. An estimated 21,000 of the 107,000 patients diag-

Levamisole made headlines in its new role in the treatment of colon cancer. The news that this drug, originally designed for a different purpose, had a new application came as no surprise to Paul Janssen, who reported such an application fifteen years ago.

sites is Dr. Oscar Vanparijs. He had worked for several years as a veterinarian in Ruanda with Dr. Marsboom. As a professor in the veterinary school at Butare, he was involved in the creation of a veterinary school for native students. Since he knew the local language, he taught parasitology and entomology, working under Dr. Thienpont. After 12 years of practical experience in Central Africa, he went to work at Janssen Pharmaceutica in 1962. He was especially involved in the creation of new parasitology research models for screening new drugs, starting from one model in chickens in 1962 to 20 models in different laboratory animals today. He succeeded Dr. Thienpont as director of parasitology in 1982.

It has been estimated that more than half of the world's population suffers from one or more types of worm infestation: hookworms, whipworms, tapeworms, and liver flukes. Some of these worms live in the human or animal gastrointestinal tract; others penetrate the skin and various organs. Some worm diseases bring extreme debilitation or death, while others are mild.

All exist as parasites on the humans or animals they infest, consuming resources that would otherwise go to making the host more energetic and healthier. The great majority of the victims are in the Third World, where the spread of these diseases is facilitated by malnutrition and inadequate sanitation. But there are many victims in North America and Europe, especially in the southern areas where both economics and climate combine to favor the spread of these parasitic diseases.

With Dr. Thienpont's arrival, the Janssen hunt for effective anthelmintics began in earnest. The technique was the usual Janssen method, involving the synthesis of new compounds and then testing the compounds for effectiveness against worms. The test animals employed were naturally infected chickens who were fed capsules containing a standard oral dose, 160 mg/kg, of each new compound. In worm investigations feces are the key indicators, so every chicken's feces were studied each day to see how many worms, if any, had been expelled.

Then on the last work day of each week, the chickens

would be sacrificed and the number of worms in the lower intestinal tracts would be counted. All through 1962 and well into 1963, the results were very discouraging. Regardless of the compound, very few worms were expelled in the feces, while a great many more worms were found alive in the intestinal tract of each chicken. A compound was needed that would cause the chickens to excrete all or almost all of their worms, leaving few or none in their bodies.

Drs. Vanparijs and Thienpont worked on these experiments. Dr. Vanparijs remembers how closely Dr. Janssen followed their tests and how eager he was to learn of their results each day. As one discouraging week followed another, Dr. Janssen's optimism did not fade. On each visit, he was not disheartened by the repeated bad news but always told Drs. Thienpont and Vanparijs, "It's good, very good. Continue on this way."

Simultaneously, Dr. Janssen was directing the program for the synthesis of new compounds. He was trying to find an effective, broad-spectrum, and nontoxic anthelmintic. In a real sense the entire program was one of random syntheses and screenings because the chemists had no leads or clues. Guided by his intuition, Dr. Janssen was convinced that the core of the desired compound would be heterocyclic, that is a ring structure containing one or more elements other than carbon. But there are an enormous number of heterocyclic compounds with which one can experiment, even using only relatively simple heterocyclic compounds as Dr. Janssen did. For a long time, as Dr. Janssen himself has confessed, "It looked as if we were climbing trees to seek fish."

However in 1963, after testing 2,721 compounds without any luck, the 2,722nd compound, R 6438, showed the desired activity in chickens. Dr. Vanparijs recalled what happened that fateful week. "At that moment, we were only two, Dr. Thienpont and I. On Monday, we treated a chicken with R 6438. Through the next several days — Tuesday, Wednesday and Thursday — we found a lot of worms in the fecal material of this chicken. It had happened many times earlier that we could find some worms in the fecal matter. But that Friday, during the autopsy on this chicken, we could not find any worms. Apparently all the worms had been expelled during the week by this substance. It was the first case that we had seen such an activity, and Dr. Paul was there to see."

But joy soon gave way to confusion and new discouragement as R 6438 was tried in other animals such as pigs, sheep, and dogs. It was found to be completely ineffective. Some thought that R 6438 should be made available even though it was effective only in chickens. Dr. Janssen vetoed that idea. There was a mystery here that needed to be solved. The idea soon emerged that R 6438 was probably a prodrug, that is, a compound which the chicken metabolized into a new compound that actually killed the worms. Other animals, it was theorized, were not capable of metabolizing R 6438 as the chicken did and hence did not produce the actual effective compound.

The metabolites of R 6438 were isolated. But synthesizing metabolites for further research was not a simple matter. Finally, the task was finished and only one of the metabolites, R 8141, proved to be active. At first sight it seemed to be an ideal candidate: It was highly potent against the important nematode group of worms, acceptably safe, very soluble in water, and seemed to work in all the main animal species.

But then new and important obstacles appeared. R 8141 was expensive to produce and tended to be unstable in water. The scientists needed to synthesize many analogues of R 8141 in the hope of finding one that had all of the original compound's virtues and none of its defects. Finally in 1964, R 8299, tetramisole, was chosen from among the alternatives as the best compound to be developed.

But the story had not ended. Tetramisole was first available as an anthelmintic in Belgium for veterinary use in 1965 and for human use in Brazil. It is actually a combination of two isomeric compounds, each the mirror image of the other, dexamisole and levamisole. Levamisole, R 12564, synthesized in mid-1966, contributes most of the anthelmintic potency observed in tetramisole. At first it was too expensive to separate the two isomers, but subsequently more efficient separation methods were found.

Levamisole ultimately became the primary anthelmintic

resulting from this long series of experiments. It turned out to be a safe, fast, and short-acting drug which is rapidly absorbed from the gastrointestinal tract, if taken orally, and from the injection site, if injected. It had required four years from the time Drs. Thienpont and Vanparijs began their screening activities until levamisole was found. Thousands of compounds had been synthesized and tested before the first success, and even after that initial morale booster, there had been many other setbacks and disappointments.

How does levamisole actually work? It causes paralysis and passive elimination of worms by interfering with the energy system of susceptible worms. It blocks the chemical reaction which gives birth to the main source of energy in worm cells, adenosine triphosphate or ATP. Throughout the ordeal of developing an effective anthelmintic Dr. Paul Janssen had remained optimistic, keeping his team at the task and personally guiding the directions in which the synthetic chemists sought to find the compound that was desired. Levamisole, the end of the line, is an excellent anthelmintic and is effective in humans as well as animals.

The story is a classic example of drug discovery. It illustrates how much failure and discouragement are a normal part of the effort. But it also illustrates that perseverance, good intuition, and a refusal to accept defeat can permit pharmaceutical researchers to make an historic and valuable contribution to medicine's armamentarium.

Dr. Marsboom, who also played a prominent role in levamisole's development, views the work as heroic. He recalled that in the early years of this project the Janssen researchers had no stable or proper experimental rooms. The autopsies were done on the same desks they wrote their reports on since their offices had to serve as laboratories. But there were no alternative working quarters. When the project was crowned with success, the hardships were worthwhile.

However, the story of the discovery of the medicinal properties of tetramisole and levamisole was not yet over. As both compounds were used increasingly, reports began surfacing of unexpected positive side effects. For example, in the small Janssen beagle breeding colony, 25 percent of the pups usually died before they were weaned. When tetramisole was used for deworming the bitches before birth, only 10 percent of the pups died before weaning. One year later, only 5 percent died.

In the Antwerp Zoo, Dr. Thienpont observed apparent cures of herpes-like viral infections in ruminants and monkeys after they received antiparasitic treatment with levamisole. In Australia, a researcher noted that calves and pigs who were doing poorly suddenly regained normal weight after treatment with tetramisole. They were apparently free of parasitic, viral, bacterial, and other infections.

Steadily the evidence mounted. Quite apart from their action against worms, tetramisole, and especially levamisole, tended to strengthen the immune systems of humans and animals, particularly those who started with impaired immune systems. Evidence also began to accumulate that in some patients whose cancers went into remission, levamisole could help extend the period of remission.

In May 1989 the United States National Cancer Institute officially designated levamisole as a Group C cancer treatment, announcing that levamisole has been shown to be potentially effective against cancer. Earlier, in February 1989, the Mayo Clinic had reported studies indicating that patients having colon cancer showed a 30-percent improvement in survival rates when treated with a combination of levamisole and the anticancer drug 5-fluorouracil. At the same time the Food and Drug Administration announced it had approved a Treatment IND which will permit physicians to use levamisole plus 5-fluorouracil as an adjuvant treatment against colon cancer beginning seven to 30 days after surgical removal of the cancer.

This breakthrough has generated considerable excitement in the medical community. Recently, a number of newspapers including *The Wall Street Journal*, *The New York Times*, and *The Washington Post* have reported on this new application for levamisole, a drug developed in 1966. But this news came as no surprise to Dr. Paul Janssen. In 1976, he published an article in *Progress Research*. It predicted that levamisole would prove to be useful against a number of different diseases by strengthening patients' immune systems.

The Janssen research in anthelmintics did not end with the successful development of levamisole. In 1968, Janssen researchers synthesized and found another effective major broad-spectrum anthelmintic, mebendazole or R 17635, known by various trade names around the world, including Vermox in the United States. Why would the same researchers who discovered tetramisole and levamisole involve themselves in the discovery of mebendazole in 1968? Why find still another compound which essentially targeted the same family of parasitic diseases as the earlier discoveries?

The immediate reason was the desire to have an anthelmintic with a wider spectrum of activity than levamisole. The target in the search for mebendazole was for an effective agent against gastrointestinal worms in sheep. When R 17635 was first tested in sheep, its excellent activity was immediately manifest. There were none of the complications that created so many obstacles on the road to finding levamisole.

But there are broader reasons for a pharmaceutical laboratory to look for another drug in the same area. First, no drug is ever perfect, and there is always hope that another drug in the same field may have properties that make it superior to the existing drug. Second is the hope that a new drug will be safer and more economical to produce and use than the existing drug. These are all valid reasons for continued research in many areas. Pharmaceutical research progresses by an incremental process in which a second-generation drug is significantly better than a first-generation compound, and a third-generation drug is significantly better than its second-generation predecessor.

There are also commercial reasons for a pharmaceutical innovator to develop new and better drugs in a given therapeutic class. These arise from the patent law which, in the United States, gives the discoverer or its licensee a monopoly on that drug's production and sale for 17 years after the patent is granted. As long as the drug is protected by patent, the innovator can begin to repay the cost of the years of research in finding and developing a drug as well as fund continuing research for new drugs. Once the patent expires, other firms can sell generic versions of the original drug. The generic drug can be priced lower because these manufacturers copy only effective and successful drugs without the investment of millions of dollars for research and development.

If a research organization is really fortunate, it may find two, three, four, or more good drugs in a particular therapeutic area in a brief period of time. It then has the option of licensing one or more of these alternative drugs to other pharmaceutical firms.

Tetramisole was synthesized in 1964, levamisole in 1966, and mebendazole in 1968. Normally that would mean that mebendazole would have a patent expiration four years later than tetramisole and two years later than levamisole. But the complexities of the developments of those two drugs were such that in actuality, in the United States, patents were granted for all three drugs between 1971 and 1972.

But that could not have been foreseen when Dr. Janssen tried to find another anthelmintic drug besides tetramisole. What he did know was that there was an orally active anthelmintic drug available, one of the earliest of the species,

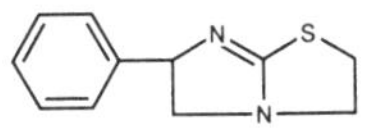

TETRAMISOLE

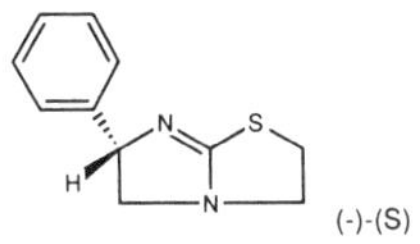

(-)-(S)

LEVAMISOLE

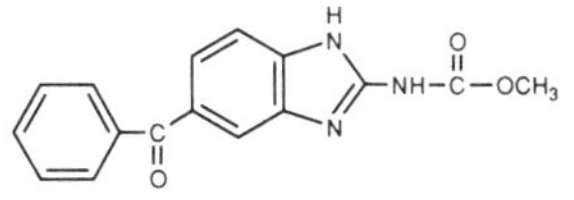

MEBENDAZOLE

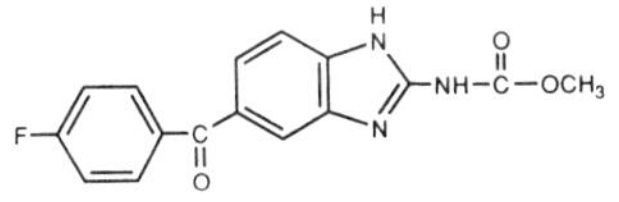

FLUBENDAZOLE

which could serve as a lead compound for the Janssen researchers. This was thiabendazole, a benzimidazole derivative which was patented by Merck & Co. in 1962. The drug is called a benzimidazole because its core is two paired rings sharing a common side, a benzene ring on the left and an imidazole ring on the right side; the imidazole ring has five sides and two vertices occupied by nitrogen atoms, separated by a carbon atom.

The challenge was to use the basic structure of thiabendazole and to synthesize variations in order to find a drug which was substantially better than thiabendazole. It was already known that thiabendazole was far from an ideal anthelmintic. Other companies had searched for derivatives or analogues of thiabendazole but without notable success. There are critics who consider this activity to be a search for "me too" drugs, which allegedly serve no purpose except quick profit for the company.

But what are found time and again are new drugs which are in many ways superior to the original compounds. Such was the case with mebendazole. It proved to be a superior anthelmintic drug, with a very wide spectrum of activity, very few safety problems, and relatively inexpensive. It is a better anthelmintic than thiabendazole and is used widely throughout the world to cure both humans and animals.

Mebendazole acts by destroying the so-called microtubules in the worm cells with the result that the worms in effect digest themselves. So the humans and animals that have been treated with mebendazole do not excrete worms. They excrete the digested remains of worms, along with the digested remains of their own food.

In a sense the discovery of mebendazole showed that the discoverers of thiabendazole had not appreciated that a useful and better anthelmintic might be made by investigating variations of the sort that led to mebendazole. If the Merck chemists had done a more thorough job, they might have been the first to find mebendazole and might have put that compound on the market rather than thiabendazole. The Janssen researchers also tried to patent a wide group of compounds similar to mebendazole. In fact, Janssen actually marketed flubendazole which, as shown, has a structure that differs from mebendazole in only one way: It has a fluorine atom at its extreme left, just beyond the benzene ring that is the extreme left-hand member of mebendazole. Flubendazole had been found to be more powerful in some respects than mebendazole, and while mebendazole caused diarrhea in pigs when given orally, flubendazole did not.

Predictably the success of mebendazole immediately attracted the attention of chemists from other pharmaceutical companies, who sought to find still other benzimidazole compounds that might be effective anthelmintics. The Janssen company, as noted, had tried to prevent that by patenting its own group of related compounds, but the ingenuity of chemists from a number of other pharmaceutical companies resulted in the discovery of other unpatented, useful compounds that could be sold in competition with mebendazole. Janssen researchers will not, nor need they, concede that any of these rivals are better than mebendazole. But with the benefit of hindsight they concede that with more work they could have obtained wider patents that would have protected mebendazole from some of the upstart competitors that appeared in subsequent years. Mebendazole has proved one of the finest products of Janssen research, serving human and animal needs on every continent and repaying the Janssen organization with revenues that permitted still more research to be carried on in the years that followed.

Dr. Janssen gave large quantities of mebendazole to the developing countries in Africa. However, local distribution systems were inadequate to provide the drug to the great majority of these populations. This situation was frustrating to Dr. Janssen and his colleagues who had developed a drug that would improve the health and quality of life for millions, and who wanted more people to benefit from it.

In more recent years, Janssen Pharmaceutica has discovered and developed other antiparasitic compounds. In early 1974 another potent anthelmintic, closantel, R 31520, was synthesized, tested, and found worthy of development. While it has a wide range of action, its particular advantage is against the liver fluke in sheep and cattle. This parasite kills animals by blocking bile ducts in the liver. In countries such as Australia, Iran, and South Africa, the liver fluke inflicts substantial economic damage.

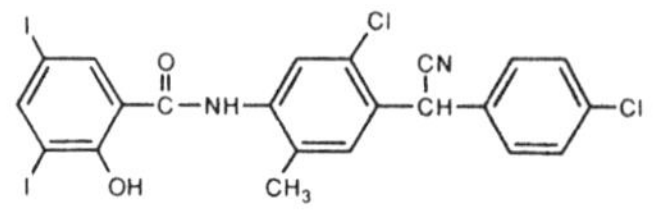

CLOSANTEL

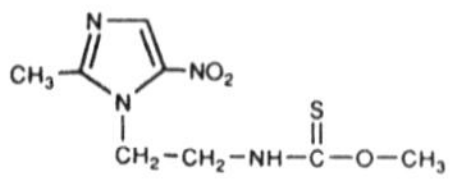

CARNIDAZOLE

Carnidazole, R 25831, an antiprotozoal drug first synthesized in 1972, is well known under its brand name Spartrix. Protozoa are one-celled organisms that can cause disease. Spartrix is effective against a family of protozoa which cause serious infections of the upper gastrointestinal system in pigeons. It is sold mainly to pigeon fanciers in Belgium, West Germany, and the Netherlands, where millions of pigeons are raised annually and the sport of pigeon racing draws many enthusiastic participants.

Chapter 8

WAGING WAR ON FUNGAL DISEASE

About a decade ago, Warner Brothers was filming the movie *The Exorcist II: The Heretic* in the southwest United States. One of the major challenges to producer John Boorman was the creation of such scenes as a Sahara Desert sandstorm which required not only huge wind machines but enough sand for a lifelike storm. Tons of sand were brought from the nearby California desert. With the sand came the fungus of valley fever disease, coccidioidomycosis. Ironically, the artificial sandstorm gave Mr. Boorman a serious case of valley fever. Despite major stars such as Richard Burton and Max von Sydow being on location, filming was halted for five weeks while Mr. Boorman recovered.

Valley fever is contracted by inhaling the causative organism, the fungus *Coccidioides immitis*, which is endemic in California's Imperial Valley, a desert turned farmland by irrigation. While valley fever and some other fungal diseases can be fatal, the most widespread of fungal infections, athlete's foot, jock itch, and ringworm, are dermatological conditions with few serious consequences.

Fungi are central characters in the eternal cycle of life and death. Fungi are the basis of our planet's ecology, permitting generation after generation of living creatures to succeed each other in a recycling of materials. Recycling on a planetary scale is what permits all kinds of life to persist over the millenia. Every living creature eventually dies and through a more or less complex process is finally reduced to its basic compounds and elements so that it can be used again for other life.

Key agents of this degradation of organic matter for reuse are bacteria and fungi. Their roles in the decomposition of organic life are the most common form of breakdown in the circular chain of life. While fungi are essential to the chain of life, environmental factors and minor changes in the delicate balance of microorganisms in humans can leave people prone to fungal infections — from the minor problem of athlete's foot to potentially lethal systemic fungal infections.

Much of the pharmaceutical and medical progress against fungal diseases since 1962 has been the result of major achievements by Janssen researchers. As a result, the generic names of these Janssen drugs — miconazole, econazole, terconazole, isoconazole, enilconazole, parconazole, ketoconazole, itraconazole, and saperconazole, among others — are known in almost all nations.

Fungi, which include yeasts, are a large group of microorganisms which normally have a filament-like or a yeast-like structure and do not have roots, stems, and leaves. They come in many sizes and colors and are capable of attacking any organic material, alive or dead. They lack the chlorophyll which gives ordinary plants and leaves their green color. This prevents fungi from synthesizing the carbohydrates and nitrogenous compounds needed for life. Hence fungi are parasitic life forms, extracting needed nutrients from living organisms or from decayed dead organisms.

In the latter case, the fungi are called saprophytes. Many of these fungi are among the simplest organisms in the world, but whether simple or complex, the fungi are found almost everywhere. All fungi reproduce nonsexually by releasing spores; some fungi can reproduce both asexually, using spores, and sexually, through the union of what are essentially male and female cells. Many fungi change their mode of reproduction from time to time depending on temperature and other shifts in the environment.

Some fungi, of course, are highly useful. A fungus was our first source of penicillin and other fungi have given us other potent antibiotics. Fungi provide us with numerous edible mushrooms, including truffles. They have also given us baker's yeast used in breads and cakes. Fungi also participate in the conversion of milk products into delectable cheeses. It is estimated that a minimum of 100,000 varieties of fungi exist.

Probably the best known fungal disease in developed countries is the nuisance ailment of athlete's foot, an external fungal infection. But when a fungus makes a successful internal invasion within our bodies, or within animals, plants, or trees, it can cripple or destroy vital organs, thus killing the unfortunate host. Since fungi normally proliferate best in heat and moisture, many severe fungal diseases are much more frequent and widespread in the tropics, particularly in the impoverished Third World countries.

Over the vastness of time, fungi have assumed many forms permitting them to live in many different environmental conditions. In the case of valley fever, the fungus has adapted to life and reproduction in a desert, illustrating the kind of flexibility with which different types of fungi adapt to almost all conditions on this planet.

People are protected against fungal disease by the same defensive immunological system that protects them against bacterial and viral diseases. Nevertheless, major fungal diseases have become a more serious problem in the developed countries of the world since World War II. Part of the reason is that modern medicines which enable people to remain alive even when their natural resistance to disease is weakened also produce conditions ideal for fungi to proliferate. Also, the widespread use of antibiotics disturbs the natural balance of the microflora and microfauna within the body, producing optimal conditions for fungal overgrowth.

Cancer patients receiving chemotherapy are among those most at risk of severe fungal infection, as are patients on intravenous medication, or with indwelling catheters or other devices which open a path from the external environment to the interior of the body. Fungi, like bacteria, are everywhere in our environment and are always available to initiate opportunistic infections. The quintessential modern plague, AIDS, is fundamentally the weakening of the natural immune system. So it is no surprise that vicious and potentially deadly systemic fungal infections are among the frequent opportunistic diseases that afflict AIDS patients.

In 1962, a group of Janssen researchers began systematic research which has brought major advances against fungal diseases. After a circuitous and unplanned research path, they made their first major antifungal discovery in 1965. Two years later they discovered far superior antifungal compounds which were made available worldwide. The Janssen discoveries of the 1970's and 1980's have proved even better than the great milestone medicines found in the 1960's.

The work against fungal diseases, like that against parasitic ailments, was partially a result of the influx of Belgian veterinarians and other scientifically oriented personnel from the Belgian Congo. One key recruit to the antifungal effort was Jan Van Cutsem, the pioneer Janssen microbiologist specializing in the search for drugs against fungal diseases. At the end of 1962, Jan Van Cutsem came to Janssen to organize a program for mycology, the study of fungi, and also bacteriology.

At that time, there was not a single appropriate screening test for these microorganisms available to Van Cutsem. It routinely took nearly six months after the synthesis of a new compound to determine its antifungal activity, if any. However, in a few short years, Jan Van Cutsem created a wide repertoire of screening tests including both *in vitro* tests in media-filled Petri dishes and tests in living cells and animals. The tests gave results in a matter of days or a few weeks at most, thus speeding up the research process enormously. Additionally, over the years Jan Van Cutsem and his associates built up one of the world's largest and most extensive collections of different fungi, providing targets against which the fungicidal properties of new Janssen compounds could be tested.

Dr. Van Cutsem worked with the organic chemist, Dr. Eric Godefroi, formerly with Parke-Davis in the United States. Noting Dr. Godefroi's interest in heterocyclic chemistry, Dr. Janssen gave him great freedom to explore the possibilities of synthesizing useful new compounds from this major branch of chemistry.

Dr. Godefroi's most important work was done with imidazoles, five-membered cyclic rings with two nitrogen atoms. It was Dr. Godefroi who made the breakthroughs that were the syntheses of econazole, R 14827, and miconazole, R 14889, both in 1967, and then of isoconazole, R 15454, which was synthesized in 1968. These discoveries helped revolutionize the treatment of human fungal diseases. Having made these historic contributions, Dr. Godefroi left Janssen Pharmaceutica to take a professorship in Holland.

Equally important was a second Janssen chemist, Dr. Jan Heeres, who has also made major contributions in this field. He worked first as Dr. Godefroi's assistant and then succeeded him as the chief of Janssen chemical research on fungicidal compounds. Born in Holland in 1941, Dr. Heeres majored in chemistry in college and then came to Janssen in 1965. Trained by Dr. Janssen and Dr. Godefroi, Dr. Heeres was the key figure in synthesizing ketoconazole, R 41400, and itraconazole, R 51211. Itraconazole contains a triazole: It has a five member cyclic structure with three nitrogens.

Ketoconazole was the first effective oral wide-spectrum antifungal drug, and its introduction greatly improved medicine's capabilities against serious fungal diseases. It is now available everywhere that modern scientific medicine is practiced. Itraconazole seems to have an even wider antifungal spectrum than ketoconazole and promises to be even more useful against the most serious systemic fungal infections.

Why were these azoles — comprised of imidazoles and triazoles — so effective against fungi? Initially, nobody knew. The actual pioneer of these compounds was an obscure chemist, D.W. Woolley, who in 1944 published his observations that the compound benzimidazole had antifungal properties. This was picked up by numerous pharmaceutical chemists. In 1967, the same year that Janssen Pharmaceutica announced the discovery of miconazole and econazole, the German pharmaceutical giant, Bayer A.G., announced that it, too, had found a highly effective antifungal drug, clotrimazole, belonging to the imidazole family, but with a distinctly different structural formula from that of the Janssen compounds.

Dr. Godefroi was given carte blanche by Dr. Janssen to explore these imidazole compounds. Curiously, the first fruits of his search had nothing to do with fighting fungi. Beginning in 1963, Dr. Godefroi synthesized two significant compounds differing slightly in their chemical structure. The first was metomidate hydrochloride or R 7315, and the second was etomidate or R 16659, available in the U.S. as Hypnomidate.

Both belonged to a new variety of short-term hypnotics useful in anesthesia, metomidate for animals and etomidate for humans. There was no expectation that hypnotic drugs would emerge from Dr. Godefroi's research. Nevertheless, it is a tribute to the Janssen screeners and screening tests that these unexpected properties were recognized. They were developed and made available for veterinary and medical use.

Dr. Marcel Janssen has summarized the chemical research philosophy of Janssen Pharmaceutica and its application in the search for antifungal drugs. "... One principle guides all our work, and that is the idea of optimization. Starting from a compound that exhibits interesting activity, we prepare derivatives and analogues, guided by what is possible chemically, by our knowledge of structure/activity relationships and by what we learn from our colleagues who are involved in screening. Our aim is to find the compound with the optimal therapeutic ratio — the drug that would be most useful to the physician.

"Starting in 1962, our early efforts at optimizing antiprotozoal activity first turned up some completely unexpected bonuses: two potent, short-acting hypnotics. Our attempts to optimize the hypnotic activity resulted in another unexpected finding: a compound without hypnotic activity but with interesting antimycotic properties."

The Janssen chemists first discovered antifungal properties when they synthesized a series of nitroimidazoles — compounds which, like the parent compound, had both an imidazole ring and a nitrogen on a side chain. These new nitroimidazole compounds did indeed control skin infections caused by the fungi known as dermatophytes, if the compounds were kept in contact with the affected skin for a prolonged period.

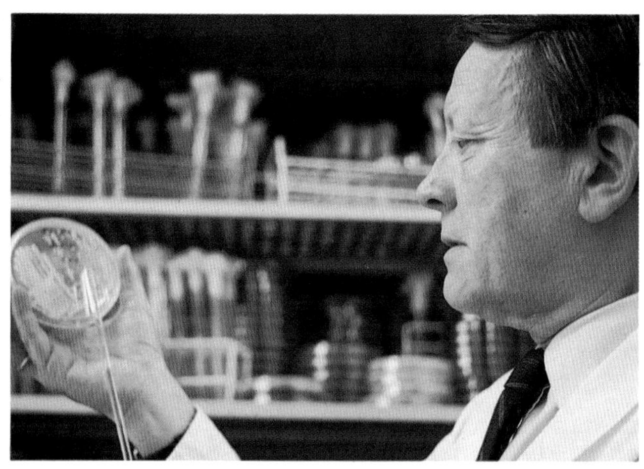

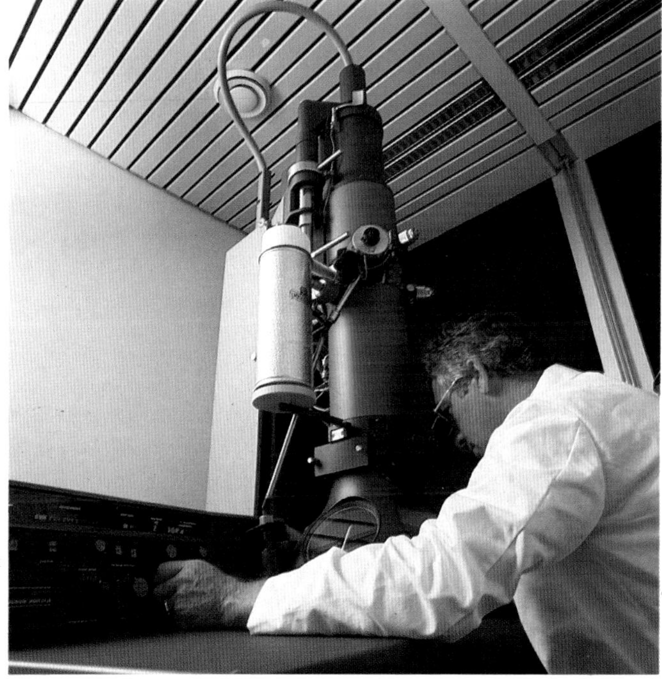

Since fungi are everywhere in our environment, the war against fungal disease is fought on many fronts. Research, aided by advancements in technology, has produced medicines that protect people, animals, and even crops from numerous diseases.

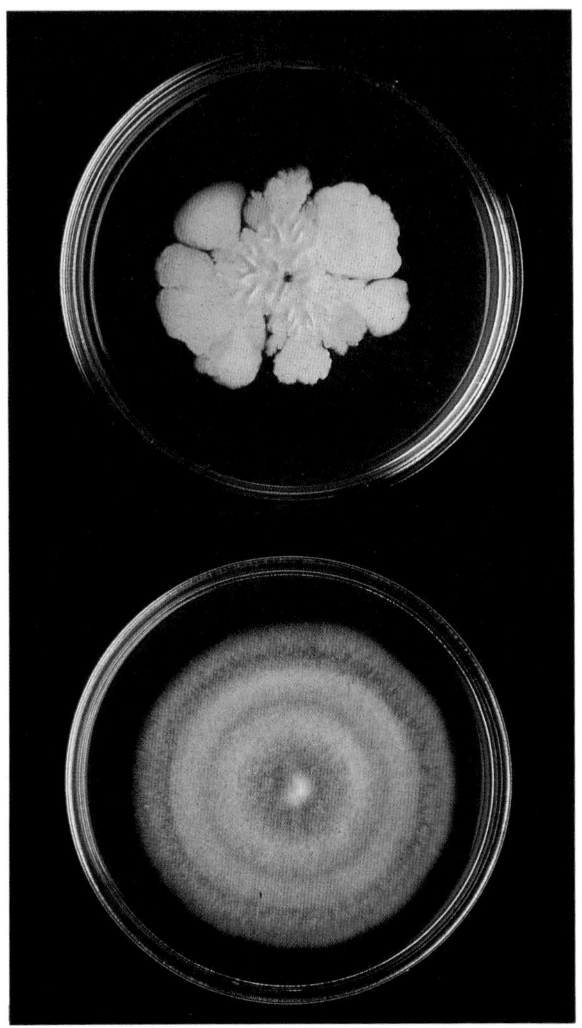

Under high magnification, the beauty of fungi belies their often harmful potential.

Unfortunately the nitroimidazoles had several serious drawbacks. First, they had objectionable odors, which patients did not welcome. Second, after these compounds were removed from the skin, the skin would have a yellow color, which also disturbed patients. Third and most serious, these compounds often irritated the skin, producing an almost intolerable burning sensation. The Janssen researchers had produced drugs which worked, but with side effects that were unacceptable to physicians and their patients.

However, in January 1965, the Janssen researchers found a new compound, which was not a nitroimidazole, did not have these side effects, and was even more effective against fungi. This compound, which became the lead for Janssen's historic contributions to antimycotic medicine, was R 10100 or etonam. Structurally, etonam is an obvious derivative of etomidate, with etomidate's CH_3 group next to the benzene ring replaced by a cyclohexane ring joined against the benzene ring.

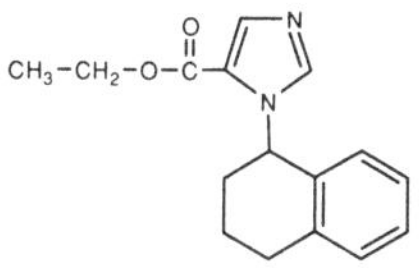

ETONAM

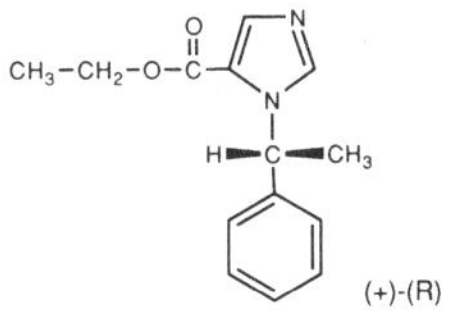

(+)-(R)

ETOMIDATE

Etonam had a curious history after its synthesis in 1965. Initially, its surprising antifungal properties were so great that it was seriously considered for human use. It was put through an extensive series of toxicological tests and then into clinical trials on patients.

In all these trials etonam's initial promise was confirmed, although a few weaknesses emerged. For example, athlete's foot is frequently caused by a variety of fungi, usually including both dermatophytes and yeasts. Etonam was effective against dermatophytes, but had no effect on the yeasts. Nevertheless etonam was such an improvement over existing antifungal drugs that its few weaknesses were accepted, and the drive to finish the testing and submit results to regulatory agencies in different countries went ahead with full steam.

But then the decision was made to abandon etonam. The reason was simple. While etonam was going through toxicological and clinical testing, the chemists had continued synthesizing new imidazole compounds, looking for still better antifungals. In the late 1960's econazole, miconazole, and isoconazole were found under the direction of Dr. Godefroi. All were superior to etonam. Dr. Heeres has estimated that it required the synthesis of about 400 compounds after the synthesis of etonam for the Janssen investigators to see that they had much better antifungal compounds than etonam.

Taking miconazole as the representative model, it consists of an imidazole ring linked by a combination of carbon, hydrogen, and oxygen atoms to two benzene rings, each of which has two chlorine atoms attached to it. The two chlorine atoms are placed on the benzene rings to slow the rate of breakdown of the compound on the skin or within the body and thus extend the period of its usefulness.

The *in vitro* and *in vivo* tests that Jan Van Cutsem ran showed that miconazole inhibited the growth of a broader range of fungi and was more effective in smaller doses than etonam. With miconazole, econazole, and isoconazole, a major new family of antifungal drugs had been discovered that were structurally similar and showed broader spectra of activity than previous compounds.

Tested *in vivo* in animals and then clinically on humans, miconazole demonstrated the same potency it had shown in earlier *in vitro* tests. But miconazole, along with econazole and isoconazole is not well absorbed when taken orally. The drug is safest and highly effective when applied topically as a cream or lotion over the infected area. Miconazole is especially effective against *Candida albicans*, a yeast that causes vaginal infections in women.

Topical miconazole has revolutionized the treatment of candidiasis. This nuisance infection is associated with the use of deodorant soaps, oral contraceptives, and broad-spectrum antibiotics and thrives in the environment created by nylon underclothing and panty hose.

Marketed as the Monistat brand in the U.S., miconazole became available to U.S. women in 1974 as once-a-day dosing in a single 14-day course of therapy. Monistat Cream offered both therapeutic and esthetic advantages over the previous standard of several repeated two-week courses of therapy with twice-a-day dosing. This was possible due to Monistat's superior efficacy and spectrum of activity. Physician and patient acceptance were overwhelming.

In the meantime, physicians in Europe were observing cure rates in dosage periods as short as three days. This led to clinical investigations of a reduced regimen in the United States. In a multicenter study to confirm these findings, investigators reported in *Obstetrics and Gynecology* in 1979 that there was no significant difference in cure rates between 7 and 14 days of Monistat cream therapy. These results confirmed the place of Monistat 7 as the treatment of choice for candidiasis.

A new dosage form, Monistat 7 Vaginal Suppositories, was introduced to the U.S. in 1982, with each suppository delivering the same amount of miconazole as one applicatorful of Monistat 7 Cream. As with previous Monistat products, this also offered esthetic advantages as well as improved dosing schedules.

Continued research in response to patients' needs led to evaluation of a Monistat suppository regimen at double the concentration of miconazole without an increase in size from the Monistat 7 Suppository. A multicenter study in the U.S. gave evidence of comparable safety and efficacy when the 3-day regimen of a single Monistat 200-mg suppository was compared to a 7-day regimen of Monistat 7 Vaginal Cream.

Currently physicians have a variety of Monistat treatment possibilities for this age-old and persistent problem. Monistat is the drug of choice for candidiasis. It has offered a major therapeutic improvement for today's women. Monistat is marketed by Ortho Pharmaceutical Co., a Johnson & Johnson company that specializes in products prescribed by gynecologists. Miconazole is also available over-the-counter as Micatin for the treatment of minor dermatological fungal infections such as athlete's foot and jock itch. These nonprescription products are offered through Ortho's Advanced Care Products Division.

In the United States, Monistat is also sold as a sterile solution for intravenous infusion for use in severe systemic fungal infections such as valley fever, candidiasis, cryptococcosis, and other similar potentially lethal fungal infections. But there may be severe side effects from the use of intravenous miconazole. Hence the FDA-approved miconazole product information stipulates that "treatment should be started under stringent conditions of hospitalization" but subsequently can be continued in ambulatory patients who are closely monitored by their physicians.

The primary educational task facing Janssen was to communicate information to physicians about the safe intravenous use of miconazole. The intravenous compound is available through Janssen Pharmaceutica's United States subsidiary whose products are mainly hospital injectables. The Janssen representatives are well suited to communicate to physicians the important safety information regarding parenteral Monistat.

But even at the moment of triumph when Janssen researchers understood how important and useful their miconazole-type antifungal drugs would be, Dr. Janssen and his associates knew that they were still far from the ultimate antifungal drug. Clearly, that would be an oral drug that could safely arrest all systemic and dermatological fungal infections. Ultimately, the ideal was a drug which could be taken as a single tablet once a day that would rid the patient of fungal infection of any kind, internal or external.

So even as miconazole, econazole, and isoconazole went into toxicological and clinical trials, Jan Heeres, Jan Van Cutsem, and their associates continued to search for an orally effective broad-spectrum antifungal drug. In general terms, they would have to come up with a compound which was absorbed more readily in the gastrointestinal tract without losing power against fungi and without any serious threat to safety.

To date, no one has discovered the ideal or ultimate antifungal drug. But almost a decade after econazole and miconazole were discovered, Dr. Heeres and his team of chemists synthesized R 41400, ketoconazole, known by the brand name Nizoral. Nizoral has many of the desirable features of the ultimate drug, but not all. It is an oral drug which is effective against a long list of fungal infections, including many yeasts. Already it has saved the lives of many whose severe systemic fungal infections could not be cured by any other available drug. But it can have one serious, though very rare, side effect: liver injury.

The group most at risk of liver injury, although it is a very small risk, consists primarily of older women, more than half of whom have a fungal infection of the nails. This seems to be an idiosyncratic reaction, but can be avoided. Clearly the risk-benefit ratio for Nizoral is heavily weighted in favor of appropriate use of the drug.

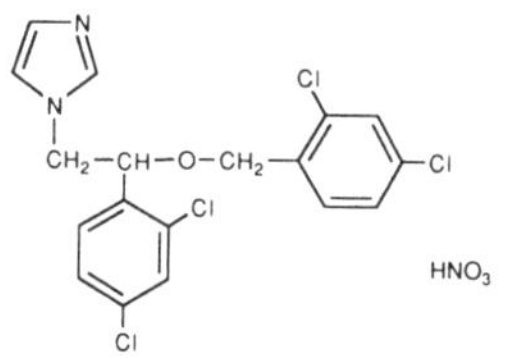

MICONAZOLE nitrate

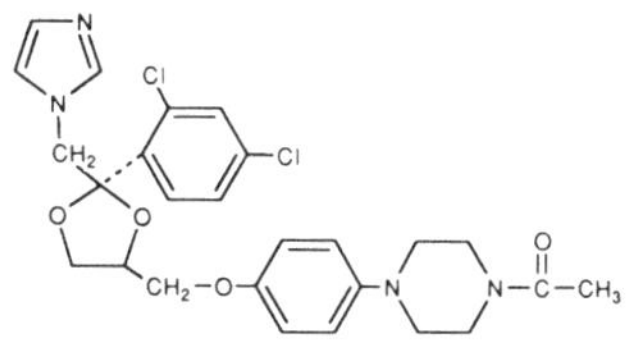

KETOCONAZOLE

Structurally, miconazole and ketoconazole are quite similar, but with some striking differences that account for the different spectrum of effectiveness between the two. Miconazole consists primarily of the imidazole ring in the upper left plus two benzene rings, each of them with two projecting chlorine atoms. Between the imidazole and the two benzene rings is a line of substituents, CH_2-CH-O-CH_2. In ketoconazole only CH_2 separates the imidazole ring from a dioxolane ring, a pentagon with two oxygen atoms at non-neighboring vertices. The dioxolane ring is directly connected to one benzene ring with two attached chlorine atoms. Immediately to the right of the dioxolane ring is a CH_2 group followed by an oxygen atom which in turn is followed by a benzene ring. But this ring does not have two chlorine atoms attached. Beyond ketoconazole's lateral benzene ring is a piperazine ring. Finally, the structural formula contains an acetyl group, a carbon atom bearing a double-bonded oxygen and a CH_3 group.

Dr. Jan Heeres makes no secret about the fact that it was an arduous hunt and test procedure that he, Dr. Janssen, and their colleagues went through before the final compound was synthesized. The dioxolane ring which is so prominent a feature of the ketoconazole molecule was added early because its virtues in an antifungal drug had been shown during the previous research which ended in the miconazole success.

One of the complications of the testing of ketoconazole, as part of the process of finally choosing it from the alternative compounds that were available, illustrates the complexities of drug research. Early *in vitro* tests were not promising until ketoconazole was tested in Eagle's minimum essential medium. Here Nizoral's great power against many fungi, especially *Candida albicans*, became evident.

Clinical testing in patients confirmed the high antifungal activity of ketoconazole. The importance attached to ketoconazole is perhaps best shown by the speed with which the FDA saw it through the tedious and time-consuming tests for safety and effectiveness. It took only three-and-one-half years after Janssen applied for permission to start clinical tests until Nizoral was approved, while the average drug takes nine years or longer to go through this gauntlet.

Many patients have been kept alive by these medicines even while their immune systems were weakening as occurs during chemotherapy for cancer patients. The advent of AIDS has created an additional population of patients who need Nizoral since their immune system deficiencies make them frequent victims of severe fungal infections.

How do miconazole, ketoconazole, and the other azole antifungal drugs exert their curative effects? Nothing was known about this matter when miconazole was first synthesized in 1967. But a great deal of information has been accumulated since, although it is unclear whether we know the full story even now.

One of the first observations made on miconazole-treated fungi with the scanning electron microscope was that the cell membranes of treated fungi had been altered compared to the membranes of normal cells. Basically, after treatment with azole antifungal drugs, the cells of fungi leak their vital contents and the cells eventually die. Why do these cell membranes become more permeable than the cell membranes of normal fungi?

The answer has to do with sterols. In mammals, including man, cell membrane permeability is governed by cholesterol, which is both manufactured in the body and ingested in food. In fungi, including yeasts, the sterol that governs cell membrane permeability is ergosterol. All of its ergosterol is produced by each fungus itself. Miconazole and ketoconazole prevent fungal cells from synthesizing ergosterol, forcing them instead to synthesize a precursor sterol, lanosterol, which is ineffective for building and regulating fungal membranes.

On the other hand azole antifungal drugs have much less impact on cholesterol formation in mammals, including humans. It takes almost 100 times as much ketoconazole to inhibit cholesterol biosynthesis in mammals as it does to inhibit ergosterol biosynthesis in the yeast *Candida albicans*. This explains why miconazole and ketoconazole can be fatal to fungi whose cells are made permeable, yet not disturb patients who continue manufacturing cholesterol as usual, and who can use cholesterol obtained from their diets.

As happens so often in science, one observation or understanding leads to another. About 1981, some doctors noted that on rare occasions male patients receiving Nizoral developed gynecomastia or enlarged breasts. Other doctors reported that this happened more often with patients battling stubborn fungal infections and receiving up to 600 mg or more of Nizoral daily. Moreover, sometimes male patients receiving these very high doses reported that they had lost their sex drive. The latter reports sometimes came from patients with swollen breasts and sometimes from patients without that symptom. Such signs of feminization of some male patients, it should be emphasized, were always reversible by lowering the dose or stopping ketoconazole administration.

These were curious side effects which clearly had to be investigated. The conclusion reached was that Nizoral aborted not only the production of the sterol fungi needed to manufacture their cell membranes, but in high doses it also aborted the production of the male hormones testosterone and the serum adrenal androgens. In effect, Nizoral was chemically castrating these patients. Since surgical castration has long been a standard treatment for cancer of the prostate, ketoconazole has given physicians an alternative to surgical procedures for victims of prostate cancer. Also treatment with ketoconazole provides the advantage of reversibility once treatment is discontinued.

All these observations suggested that Nizoral or its metabolites might be a useful drug for patients with prostatic cancer. A great deal of research has since been invested toward that objective. Janssen scientists and physicians are intensively studying the action of R 75251, which blocks the production of androgens and therefore may be useful against cancer of the prostate. R 75251 is not derived directly from ketoconazole but it was synthesized in the research effort initiated when the potential action of ketoconazole against prostatic cancer was realized.

The mere possibility that a drug developed for fungal infection may yet give rise to an important anticancer medication emphasizes again that the human body is a highly integrated organism. Both physicians and pharmaceutical researchers must always be looking for the unexpected phenomenon that may provide clues to objectives far different from those sought when a given research project begins.

In 1980 Janssen chemists synthesized another major candidate, itraconazole, R 51211. This new class of oral wide-spectrum antifungal drugs opens new perspectives for even better drugs in the future. Itraconazole has been tested extensively *in vitro*, in animals, and in the clinic. It is clearly more potent in various fungal infections than either miconazole or ketoconazole. It can cure some fungal diseases, notably aspergillosis, that neither of the latter can usually cure.

Itraconazole is, in fact, the first orally active antifungal to be effective against aspergillosis; it also produces remarkably good results against sporotrichosis, meningeal cryptococcosis, and in most pheohyphomycoses. And it seems to have a high degree of safety. It promises to be a major weapon against the most invasive fungi that plague AIDS patients and others with impaired immune systems.

Terazole (terconazole), the first of a new generation of antifungals, is one of the most recent Janssen compounds to be introduced in the United States. Its mode of action is both innovative and efficient for the local treatment of vaginal candidiasis or yeast infections. While terconazole is not as broad-spectrum as miconazole, it is highly effective against *Candida.*

The FDA approved Terazole as a 7-day regimen of a cream formulation in late 1987 and as a 3-day suppository regimen in mid-1988. The product has an outstanding cure rate both clinically and microbiologically, with most patients reporting relief by day three. Thus Janssen research has provided yet another improved treatment for this common gynecological problem.

Recent efforts have brought about a potentially superior compound, R 66905, saperconazole. It is now under careful study. Saperconazole is superior to itraconazole in fighting aspergillosis infections. It can be administered safely and effectively intravenously. No other Janssen antifungal drug can be used so effectively against major internal fungal diseases.

Fungi also attack other life forms besides humans. They attack plants, trees, animals, stored vegetables, fruit and grain, and even cut wood used in construction. Janssen Pharmaceutica has made major contributions to the fight against fungal damage in these cases — damage that annually amounts to a huge economic loss.

In 1971, R 23979 was synthesized. It is the only Janssen compound that has two generic names. As enilconazole, it is known widely among livestock and chicken breeders, bird fanciers and veterinarians. As imazalil, it is known and esteemed highly by farmers and managers of warehouses that store farm products from grain to citrus fruits and apples. In both categories, R 23979 fights fungal infections that would otherwise inflict huge losses on agricultural production and harm consumers who use animal and vegetable products of every kind.

Meanwhile the hunt for more effective antifungals continues at Janssen. The early pioneers Jan Van Cutsem and Jan Heeres still work under Dr. Janssen and are training a new generation of chemists, microbiologists, and other scientists in the war against fungi. Their work will benefit the health of people, crops, and domestic animals, and help raise the standard of living for many people. Perhaps this wealth of antifungal knowledge will soon produce a major new chemotherapeutic drug for cancer of the prostate. The hope exists daily with the men and women at Janssen Pharmaceutica that their labors will produce drugs that will protect the health of people around the world as well as provide better treatment and improved quality of life when disease does strike. Their success is ultimately humanity's gain.

Chapter 9

MENDING LINKS IN THE DIGESTIVE CHAIN

As astronauts float in the very low gravity of their space capsules, the control of their bowel movements is a point of concern. It is not only a matter of health but an important element in the safe and accurate execution of their mission responsibilities. Astronauts on prolonged flights, including the Apollo flight to the moon, faced this health issue. Unknown at the time, the doctors caring for the astronauts used the Janssen-discovered antidiarrheal drug, diphenoxylate, R 1132. The drug proved most efficent even in this special use.

Diphenoxylate's role in the space program need not surprise us. Of all the important Janssen drugs available to physicians the world over, none have reached and helped more people than the Janssen antidiarrheal compounds: Lomotil (diphenoxylate) or R 1132 and Imodium (loperamide) or R 18553.

More than four billion tablets of diphenoxylate, whose brand names in various countries also include Reasec, Diarsed, and Retardin, have been taken by patients over the past 30 years. In recent years, Imodium, which was discovered in 1969, thirteen years after diphenoxylate, has become more popular. In 1988, a liquid form of Imodium was approved for over-the-counter use in the United States, an indication of the high safety profile of this compound.

Diarrhea is not a negligible ailment, though its frequency in all countries invites the contempt bred by familiarity. Today diarrhea is discussed publicly, most often in connection with children in the Third World where incredibly high numbers of children die needlessly of diarrhea each year. Diarrhea is also very familiar in the developed countries. Frequently, diarrhea is caused by an infection or it may result from some contaminated food or polluted water.

Such serious chronic diseases as ulcerative colitis and spastic colitis have diarrhea among their most frequent symptoms. Surgery of the intestinal tract is often followed by diarrhea. Traveler's diarrhea, memorialized by such names as Montezuma's revenge and Delhi belly, is a frequent phenomenon in this era of mass tourism when each year vacationers fly thousands of miles from home, often to areas with major differences in climate, food, and water. Shock or psychological stress may also induce diarrhea as with many infantrymen when they first experience combat.

Diarrhea is very rarely a fatal disease in the developed world, although it often makes its victims' lives miserable. Understandably, victims of significant, sustained diarrhea eagerly seek a medicine that will quickly end their discomfort. Often that medicine has been one of the two Janssen synthetic antidiarrheal drugs.

When water and food travel down the esophagus to the stomach, they are digested to a pulpy fluid called chyme. Small amounts of chyme are soft enough to be transferred by peristaltic movements to the small intestine, consisting of the duodenum, the jejunum, and the ileum. It continues its peristaltic progress through the gastrointestinal tract. The further the chyme goes, the more it is broken down into simple nutrients which are absorbed into the blood stream.

The small intestine joins the large intestine, or colon, at the cecum. What is left of the digested food passes through the large intestine. Additional nutrients are absorbed with a massive reabsorption of large quantities of fluids, secreted in the gastrointestinal tract, which have played a major role in the digestive process. Finally, in a normally functioning digestive system, the remaining undigestible portion of the chyme, mixed with only a small quantity of fluid, is excreted through the rectum as well-formed stool.

Diarrhea of many forms results when something has gone wrong with the process along the complex digestive chain. Precisely because diarrhea has many causes, it would be a Herculean task to try to diagnose and treat each cause, assuming even that all causes of diarrhea are treatable.

What the Janssen synthetic antidiarrheal drugs have done is to make it possible, in the great majority of cases, to deal with the symptoms of diarrhea: the excessive frequency and liquid consistency of stools and the pain that often accompanies diarrhea. Once the patient is comfortable, chances are very good that the body itself will soon correct the cause of the diarrhea. Only in a small fraction of cases does the actual cause of diarrhea have to be ascertained and, if possible, treated. Diarrhea is, of course, only a symptom, but it is a distressing symptom which can be addressed while the natural recuperative forces of the body work to regain good health.

People over 40 years of age are likely to remember that if, as children or adults, they had diarrhea which caused them to consult a physician, the frequent remedies offered before 1960 were the opiates: tincture of opium and paregoric. These once-standard remedies took advantage of the fact that among the properties of opium and its derivatives is the ability to stop diarrhea. But although physicians prescribed the opiates, they did so with some misgivings. They knew that opium and its derivatives could create addiction, a problem far more serious than the original diarrhea.

Moreover, many opium derivatives have undesirable central nervous system effects such as stupor and excessive sedation. Many a physician must have mused in the past about what a blessing it would be if somebody could separate the antidiarrheal property of opium from the addictive properties. Dr. Paul Janssen and his colleagues accomplished just that.

In 1956 diphenoxylate was discovered. Two years earlier, Dr. Janssen had discovered isopropamide, R 79, an antispasmodic. Diphenoxylate emerged as the addition of isopropamide and meperidine. The left-hand side of the diphenoxylate molecule is a simplified version of the isopropamide molecule, while the right-hand side of the diphenoxylate molecule is the meperidine molecule. But the actual discovery process wasn't that simple. Dozens of possible compounds were synthesized, most of them tested and rejected. A few were tested and used as the basis for still other compounds that came closer to what was desired. Finally, the molecule diphenoxylate was synthesized.

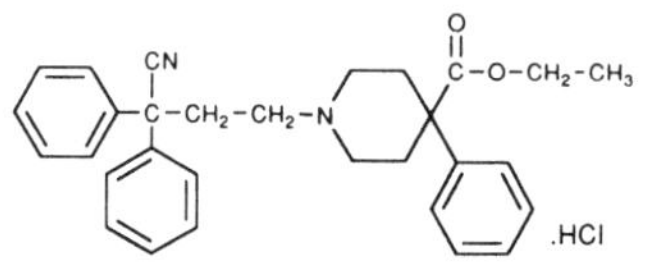

DIPHENOXYLATE hydrochloride

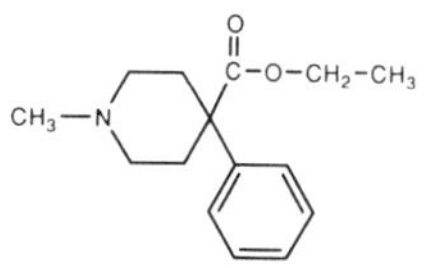

MEPERIDINE

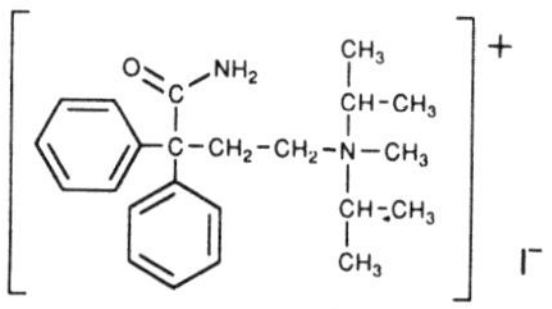

ISOPROPAMIDE iodide

By present standards, the techniques Dr. Janssen and his colleagues had available in the mid-1950's to test *in vivo*, or in animals, whether a compound was an antidiarrheal drug were extremely primitive. A mouse was given an injection of the compound being tested and also fed a meal of charcoal mixed with something that would make it relatively palatable. After a fixed period of time, the mouse would be autopsied. How much of the length of the digestive tract had the charcoal traveled? Had the charcoal reached the juncture of the small and large intestine?

In effect, these tests indicated the extent to which the compound being tested had slowed down the movement of material being processed. In retrospect, it is clear that these tests were really tests of the constipating effect of the compounds being studied. But the assumption was that if constipation was the opposite of diarrhea, then a compound capable of causing constipation would stop diarrhea.

In the case of diphenoxylate, this assumption proved true. Diphenoxylate became the first major international drug success achieved by Janssen Pharmaceutica. Within a few years, the drug was available in almost all countries. Its success allowed the Janssen enterprise to broaden its research staff and facilities.

There was, however, one hitch that threatened to delay the availability of the drug. The compound's structural relation to meperidine, a synthetic morphine, was obvious to every chemist. Did that mean that diphenoxylate would be an addicting drug? Dr. Janssen pointed out that the central nervous system effects of diphenoxylate were minimal. Tests were done and no signs emerged of a euphoric effect that might suggest future addiction or abuse. But not all observers were convinced.

Finally a solution was found. In every formulation, whatever amount of diphenoxylate was included, there would be one-percent atropine sulfate included, on the theory that this would discourage deliberate overdosage. To this day the official patient information insert required by the FDA includes this admonition: "Lomotil is not an innocuous drug and dosage recommendations should be strictly adhered to, especially in children."

But almost thirty years of experience with diphenoxylate in all parts of the world have shown no significant evidence that it leads to addiction or other abuse. Dr. Janssen's belief that the supposed danger was exaggerated seems to have been thoroughly vindicated by the test of time.

Diphenoxylate is, strictly speaking, a constipating drug. Depending upon the quantity administered, it stops peristalsis in the intestinal system for a time, or slows down peristalsis so that, where required, there will be only one defecation a day. This property of diphenoxylate explains its use in the U.S. National Aeronautics and Space Administration (NASA) programs. Astronauts cannot necessarily stop what they are doing at any point and go to the bathroom. According to Dr. Charles Berry, in a comment written while he was medical chief of the United States astronaut program, diphenoxylate was chosen to "assist in avoiding inflight defecation when necessary."

Between 1956 and 1968 the research staff at Janssen Pharmaceutica synthesized and tested more than 14,000 new compounds looking for, among other things, an even better antidiarrheal drug than diphenoxylate. What they found in 1968 was diphenoxin, R 15403, brand name Dioctin, which was the most active metabolite of diphenoxylate. Diphenoxin was found to be about five times as potent, per unit weight, as diphenoxylate, with the advantage of fewer central nervous system side effects.

But a year or so after diphenoxin was discovered, Janssen chemists found a much better antidiarrheal, loperamide, R 18553, which is known in the United States as Imodium. Dr. Janssen wrote in 1976, "In 1969, when a new method for the synthesis of basic amides ... was found, interest in the field of antidiarrheal drugs was revived. It was found that several members of the new series, but in particular loperamide, chemically related to the classic neuroleptic haloperidol ... were not only more potent and longer acting than diphenoxylate in animals and in man, but surprisingly free of morphine-like or other central nervous system effects, even at high-dose levels.

"A goal of completely separating antidiarrheal and central nervous system activity had been realized. After five years of extensive pharmacological, toxicological, biochemical and clinical investigations, loperamide was available in 1974 in 2-mg capsules and is at present clearly the drug of choice for the symptomatic treatment of diarrhea."

The structural formulas of diphenoxylate, diphenoxin, loperamide, and loperamide N-oxide provide many similarities as well as some key differences. These compounds have two benzene rings at the left which are connected by a $C\text{-}CH_2\text{-}CH_2$ chain to a piperidine ring which is in turn connected to a benzene ring.

Diphenoxylate and diphenoxin have only one difference in structural formula. A group of atoms attached to the piperidine ring in diphenoxylate is the rather complex combination $COOC_2H_5$. In diphenoxin, that group of atoms becomes simply $COOH$. In all other respects, the two molecules are identi-

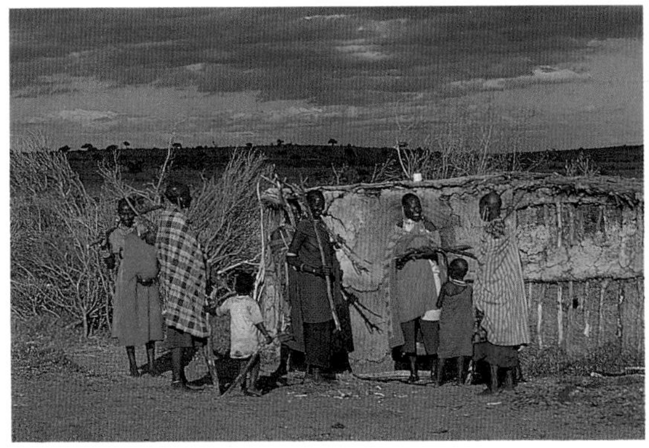

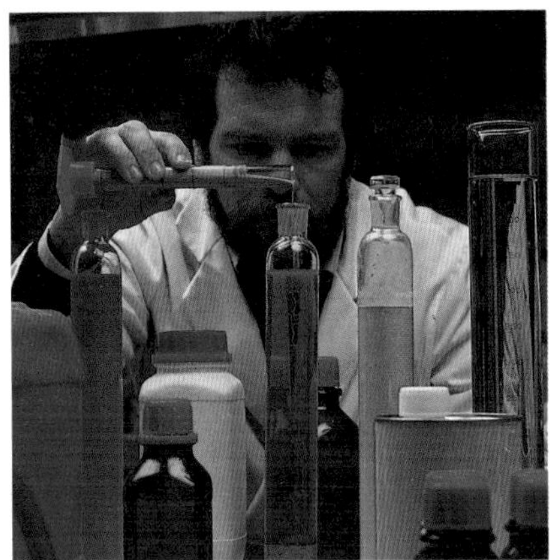

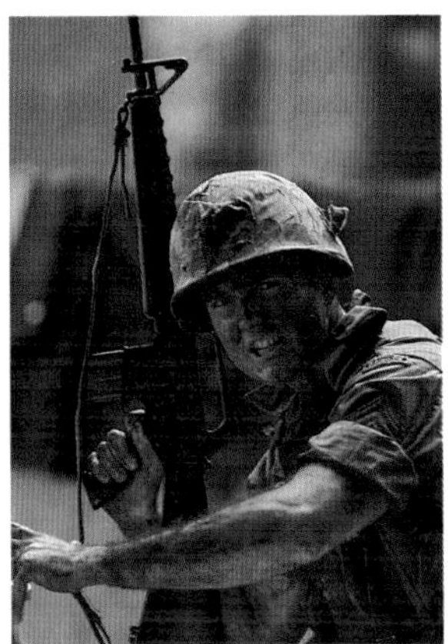

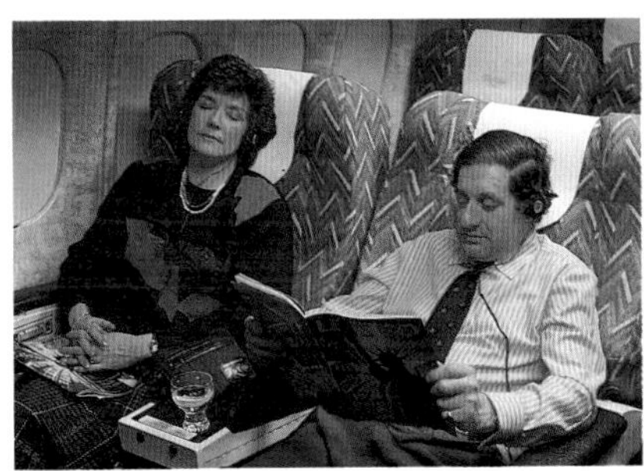

To people in Third World countries, diarrhea can be fatal. International travelers consuming food and water, or soldiers under the stress of combat can also experience this disorder. Scientists are constantly seeking better medicines to strengthen the weak link in the digestive chain.

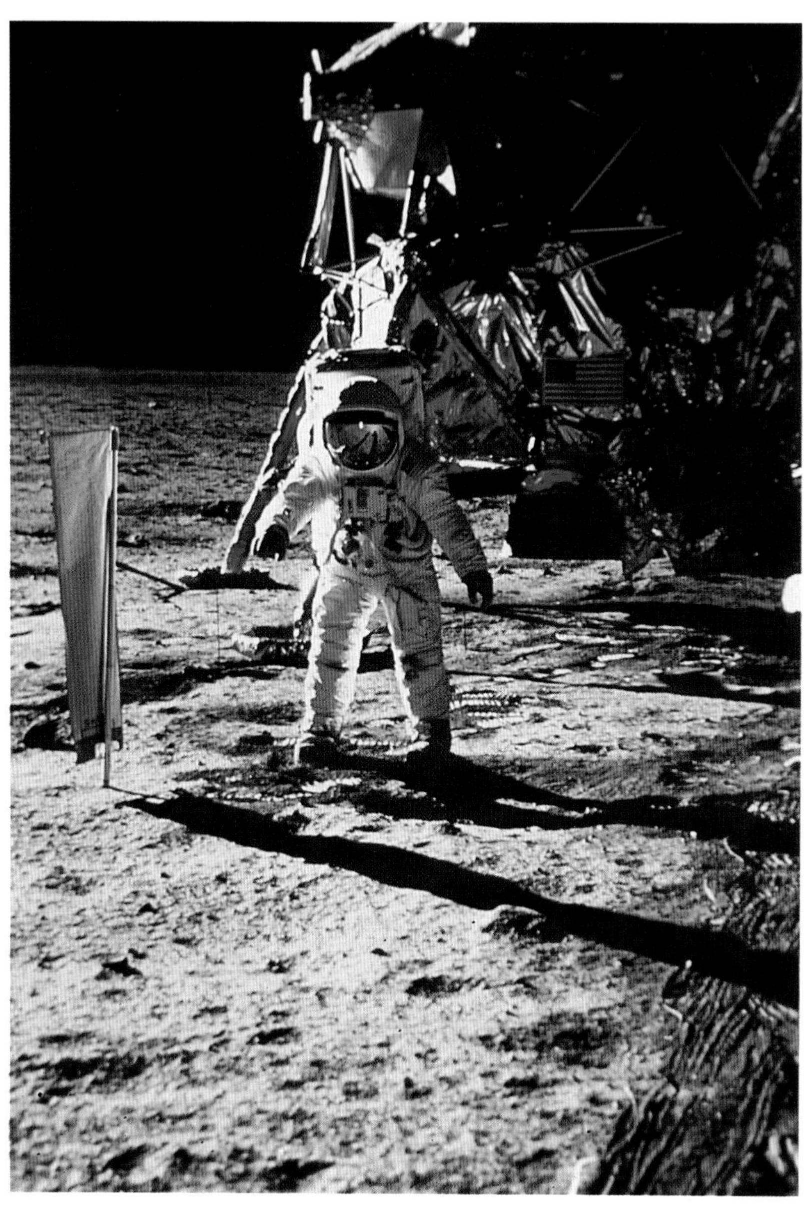

The Apollo astronauts were concerned with controlling bowel movements in their long flight to the moon. Consequently diphenoxylate, a Janssen drug, played a role in the lunar mission.

cal, including the cyano group (CN) above the carbon in the chain connecting the left-hand pair of chemical rings with the right-hand pair.

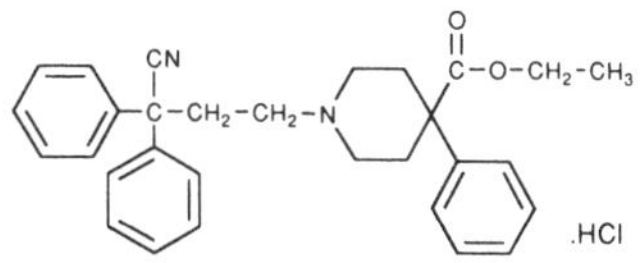

DIPHENOXYLATE hydrochloride

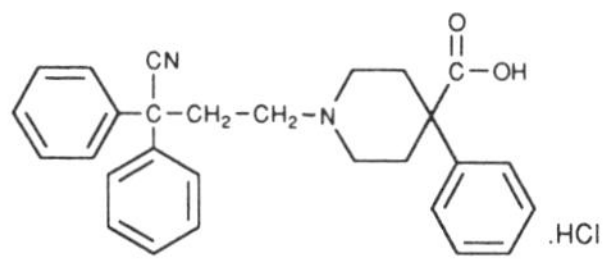

DIPHENOXIN hydrochloride

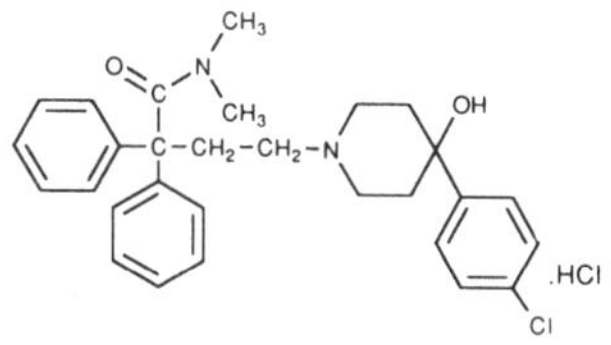

LOPERAMIDE

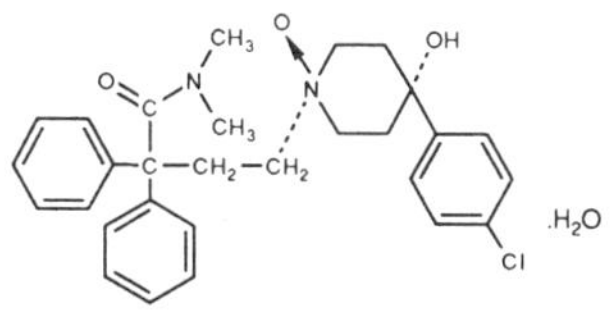

LOPERAMIDE oxide

In loperamide, each of the two groups of atoms described immediately above as attached to the piperidine ring in diphenoxylate and diphenoxin respectively are replaced by the simple hydroxyl radical while the right-hand benzene ring has a terminal chlorine attached.

But the real difference in chemical structure and in biological action between the two earlier antidiarrheals and loperamide presumably comes from the replacement of the cyano group by a dimethyl carboxamide complex combination of oxygen, carbon, nitrogen, and hydrogen. Just why that difference makes loperamide so much more superior to its two predecessors is unknown.

How did the pharmacologists, working under the leadership of Janssen long-time director of pharmacology, Carlos Niemegeers, prove that loperamide was an effective antidiarrheal drug with practically no central nervous system effect?

They did it by using two *in vivo* tests. One proved that loperamide was an effective antidiarrheal by showing that it halted diarrhea in rats who were given castor oil. This is a direct test of a drug's ability to stop diarrhea, rather than an indirect test pointing primarily to a drug's power to produce constipation as had been true of the charcoal meal test used originally in the late 1950's with diphenoxylate. Loperamide could stop diarrhea in 50 percent of a group of rats given a standard dose of castor oil when loperamide was administered in as small an amount as 0.15 mg per kilogram of a rat's weight.

As a measure of central nervous system activity, the pharmacologists tested for the analgesic effect of loperamide by using the tail withdrawal test. It was found that loperamide had to be administered at a very high, near lethal dose level to show any analgesic effect, but it had the ability to stop diarrhea when administered in a very low dose. Thus the tests showed that loperamide had virtually none of the connection between antidiarrheal action and addictive or other central nervous system properties usually found in opium derivatives.

It is significant that Imodium (loperamide) has no atropine content, nor does the package information material have any warning such as that on diphenoxylate. Instead the FDA-approved patient package insert states, "Abuse: A specific clinical study designed to assess the abuse potential of loperamide at high doses resulted in a finding of extremely low abuse potential. Additionally after years of extensive use, there has been no evidence of abuse or dependence."

In 1988, the FDA ruled that Imodium (loperamide) may be sold as an over-the-counter drug with no prescription required. This change in status reflects Imodium's superior safety profile and very low potential for abuse. Loperamide may not be the end of the line of the successful Janssen synthetic antidiarrheal drugs. In 1983, compound R 58425, called loperamide N-oxide, was synthesized, and this appears to have some advantages over loperamide in certain specific situations. Loperamide N-oxide's structural formula differs from that of loperamide only in having an oxygen atom linked to the nitrogen of the piperidine ring. Loperamide N-oxide seems to be a prodrug of loperamide. When loperamide N-oxide is administered orally to a living organism, it is metabolized in the presence of intestinal contents to loperamide and then has the antidiarrheal effect.

The major rationale for developing loperamide N-oxide was to reduce the risk of intoxication after acute overdosing. Indeed, while loperamide has been found both safe and efficacious in very young infants, this has been true only in well-nourished hospitalized children who had supplementary measures such as hydration available for their treatment as needed.

But in malnourished infants and other infants in less than optimal condition, loperamide may be less safe because of accidental excessive uptake into the circulation. In the case of loperamide N-oxide, high plasma levels are unlikely to occur since metabolic conversion of the N-oxide to loperamide occurs mainly in the gut and the gut wall, where it has its effects and where it will be metabolized into inactive compounds before reaching the systemic circulation.

This reasoning has now been confirmed by clinical trials. These have shown that loperamide N-oxide is not only safer than loperamide, but also more effective.

Chapter 10

NEW HOPE FOR DIGESTIVE DISORDERS

Andre Reyntjens, M.D., former coordinator of international clinical testing and now vice chairman of the Janssen Research Council, likes to tell this story. In 1974, Dr. Paul Janssen sat down with some of his key people and expressed dissatisfaction with the lack of progress in gastroenteric drugs. Aside from the antidiarrheals, the company had only one relevant drug, the antispasmodic drug isopropamide, R 79, which had been discovered 20 years earlier. Couldn't isopropamide be improved?

Dr. Reyntjens spoke up. It would be difficult to improve on the existing antispasmodic drug. He suggested that the Janssen scientists look to the field of drugs affecting gastrointestinal motility. There was an existing drug, metoclopramide (brand name Reglan in the United States), but it had some undesirable neuroleptic or central nervous system side effects. Dr. Reyntjens believed that this area of drug research would provide better results.

Dr. Janssen considered the idea and agreed that it was a viable avenue of research. Dr. Janssen believed that success in research was better achieved when researchers followed their own instincts. So the five-minute meeting ended with a decision that set in motion the events which would spawn a major drug, domperidone, R 33812. Years later, Dr. Janssen said, "The decision was not quite that simple." Nevertheless, the story reflects the confidence Dr. Janssen had in his staff.

Dr. Reyntjens had been Dr. Janssen's classmate in medical school. After graduation, he went into medical practice in Antwerp and for eight years bore a heavy load of hospital and ambulatory medicine, caring for thousands of patients. The many hours of work made him a stranger to his children. So he eventually sought an alternative career. His daily hands-on contact with patients proved invaluable in his new position in the pharmaceutical industry. He joined Janssen Pharmaceutica in 1969, when there were two medical doctors engaged full-time in conducting clinical trials.

Dr. Janssen suggested that Dr. Reyntjens turn his attention to clinical trials abroad. Until that time, trials on Janssen drugs outside Belgium had been done by licensees or by drug importers. But Dr. Janssen was aware of the need to improve the quality of clinical trials conducted on Janssen drugs abroad and to institute better control over them. Today, the Janssen international clinical trials staff has several dozen members representing subsidiary companies on all continents. They work with literally hundreds of physicians who conduct clinical trials. Dr. Reyntjens' arrival was the beginning of that organization.

What Dr. Reyntjens had in mind in that brief meeting in 1974 when he told Dr. Janssen about the need for motility drugs — also called prokinetic drugs — was the problem of nausea and vomiting. Although the issue had never been addressed in medical literature, Dr. Reyntjens was fascinated by the analogy between upper gastrointestinal malfunction in patients with dyspepsia and that associated with nausea.

Dyspeptic patients may have documented decreased esophageal peristalsis and an incompetent lower esophageal sphincter that result in reflux of gastric contents into the esophagus. They may also show a slack stomach and insufficient width of the duodenum into which the stomach empties, hindering normal outflow of the stomach's contents. But direct measurement during nausea shows a constricted duodenum, spasm of the exit from stomach to the duodenum, and often an open passage between the esophagus and the stomach. So vomiting or emesis might well be causally related to gastrointestinal dysmotility.

Emesis, or vomiting, probably has as many causes in the

upper gastrointestinal tract as diarrhea has in the lower tract. Both are symptoms of digestive distress. But medical progress has also contributed to this condition. Many drugs used to combat cancer, for example, tend to produce nausea and vomiting. If these distressing symptoms are not stopped, the treatment may have to be discontinued. The patient who might have been cured or had his life extended remains ill because the nausea and vomiting could not be curbed.

It had already been noted that antipsychotic drugs such as haloperidol tended to stop vomiting as well as to successfully address psychotic symptoms. But it seems impractical to ask a patient to take a potent antipsychotic drug, with all its potentials for side effects, in order to stop vomiting.

The problem was how to separate the two effects: antiemetic and antipsychotic activity. When Dr. Janssen gave his approval in that brief meeting, Dr. Reyntjens committed himself and his research colleagues to finding a drug which stopped or prevented vomiting without producing the central nervous system effects of an antipsychotic drug.

Metoclopramide, which was discovered by French scientists in the 1950's, separated the antipsychotic and antivomiting effects imperfectly. The warning contained in the package information insert authorized by the FDA for metoclopramide states:

"Extrapyramidal symptoms, manifested primarily as acute dystonic reactions, occur in approximately 1 in 500 patients treated with metoclopramide. These occur more frequently in children and young adults and are even more frequent at the higher doses used in the prophylaxis of vomiting due to cancer chemotherapy. These symptoms may include involuntary movements of limbs and facial grimacing, torticollis, oculogyric crisis, rhythmic protrusion of tongue, bulbar type of speech, trismus, or dystonic reactions resembling tetanus ... Parkinsonism as well as rare persistent dyskinesias have been reported."

But there was a clue to the separation of the antipsychotic effect of a neuroleptic-type drug from the antivomiting or antiemetic action. For some neuroleptics, there was an antiemetic effect with only one-fifth of the dose needed to produce antipsychotic action. Dr. Reyntjens had noted that in some of the later neuroleptic drugs discovered by Janssen, the antiemetic action was obtained with only one-fifteenth the dose needed for antipsychotic activity.

Why not follow up that lead and look for neuroleptic-type compounds in which the dose for antiemetic activity was a very great deal less than the dose required for antipsychotic activity? The rationale was that undesirable side effects, such as those outlined for metoclopramide, appear when a drug is used whose antiemetic dose is too close to its antipsychotic dose. The adverse reactions actually stemmed from the antipsychotic activity of the drug.

Dr. Reyntjens and Dr. Janssen discussed these ideas with the Janssen staff of chemists and the pharmacologists. The strategy was to synthesize a number of neuroleptic-type drugs and find which chemical structure alteration gave the greatest separation of antiemetic and antipsychotic action; that is, which structure would make the antiemetic dose the smallest fraction of the antipsychotic dose. The next step was to find a drug whose antiemetic dose is such a tiny fraction of the antipsychotic dose that, for all practical purposes, the drug no longer has neuroleptic activity.

That strategy yielded domperidone. It is a drug that produces effective antiemetic action at a dose which is 1/250th of the lowest dose required to get an antipsychotic effect. About 100 compounds were synthesized and studied before domperidone was found, a remarkably small number of compounds in a short period of time.

Pharmacologically, the neuroleptics are dopamine antagonists. Dopamine is a well-known neurotransmitter which also operates in the stomach and intestinal tract. Dopamine antagonists block dopamine receptors in the brain and elsewhere, and thus mitigate the effects of the excess of dopamine that apparently exists in the brains of psychotic individuals. It is this blocking of dopamine receptors that is also responsible for the antiemetic effects of neuroleptic drugs.

The blood-brain barrier operates as though it were a membrane-like sheath that protects the brain against most compounds that course through the human body. A drug or

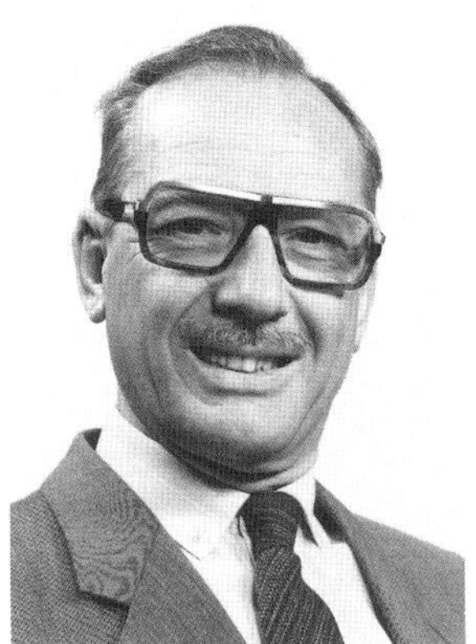

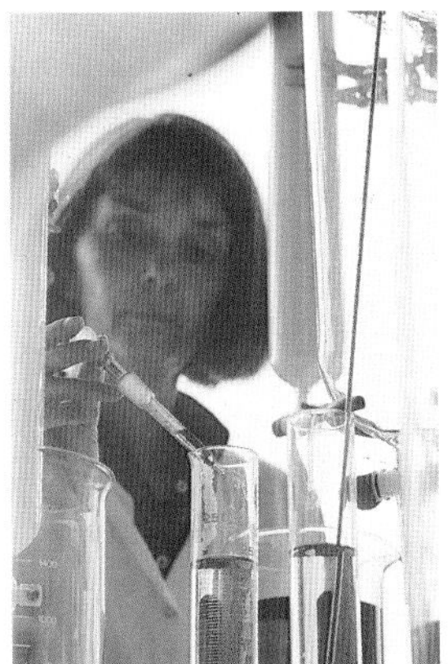

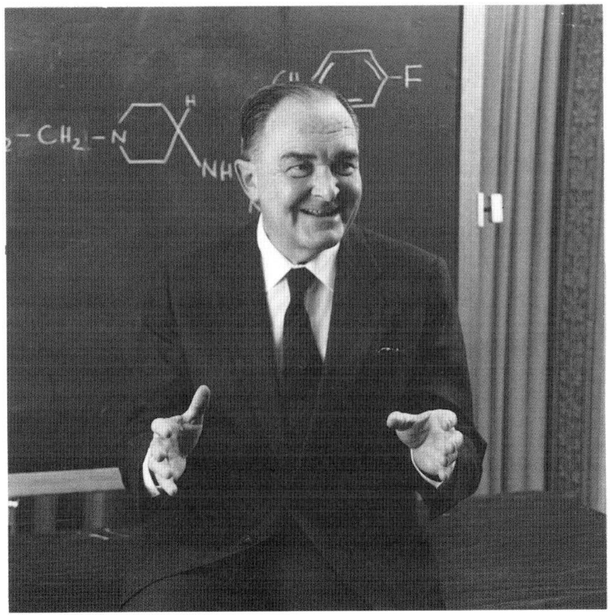

Dr. Andre J. Reyntjens (top left) took his research in an unexpected direction. A new family of motility drugs (prokinetic drugs) to treat digestive disorders was discovered. Dr. Paul Janssen has always encouraged scientists to research problems that interest them. "We try to build research around people."

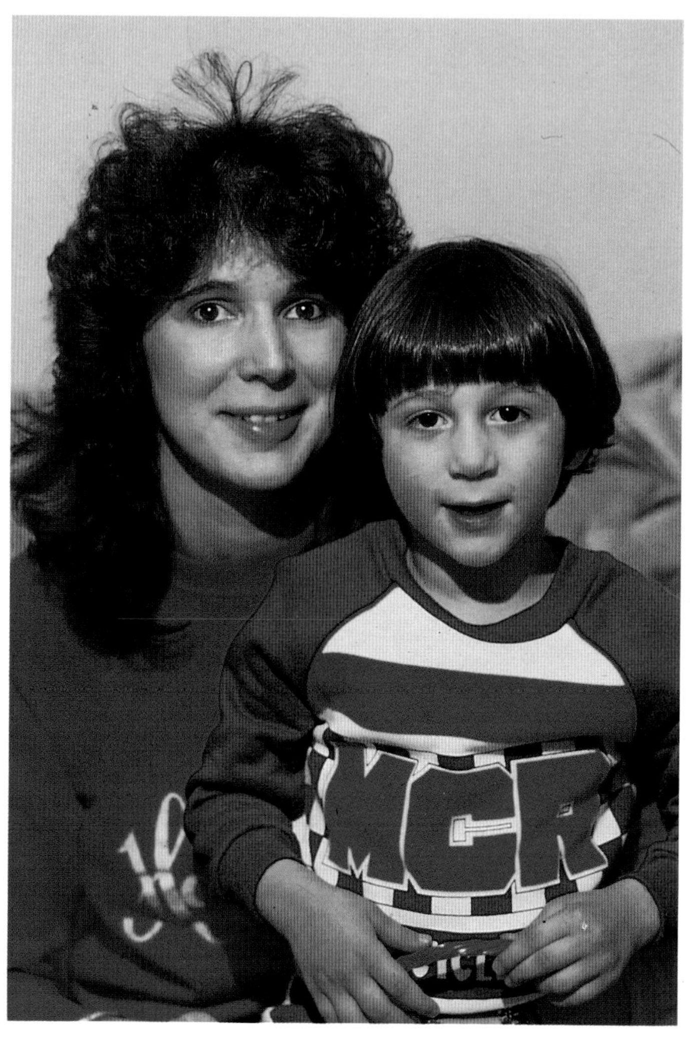

Patrick Spinella, born with a rare intestinal disease, underwent seven operations and wore a fitted backpack that pumped nutritional formula into him. With hope fading and his medical bills exceeding $100,000, doctors learned of a new Janssen drug called Prepulsid. It saved Patrick's life.

other compound can only affect the brain if it passes through the blood-brain barrier. Obviously, to act against psychoses, neuroleptics have to be capable of penetrating the blood-brain barrier and blocking dopamine receptors in the brain.

Emesis is controlled by a portion of the brain called the chemoreceptor trigger zone located just outside the blood-brain barrier. So the problem of separating the antipsychotic effects from the antiemetic effects of a neuroleptic-type drug can be stated this way: find a drug that will not pass through the blood-brain barrier, or will pass through it only to a very small extent. That compound will be antiemetic because it does what is needed outside the blood-brain barrier. Its antipsychotic activity, if any, will be brief since it either cannot penetrate the blood-brain barrier or does so very poorly.

The blood-brain barrier is most easily breached by lipophilic drugs or compounds that dissolve easily in fats. The blood-brain barrier is very difficult or impossible to breach if a compound is hydrophilic or very easily soluble in water. This knowledge was critical in synthesizing domperidone. As a result, domperidone substantially reduces nausea and vomiting with little risk of the side effects of metoclopramide.

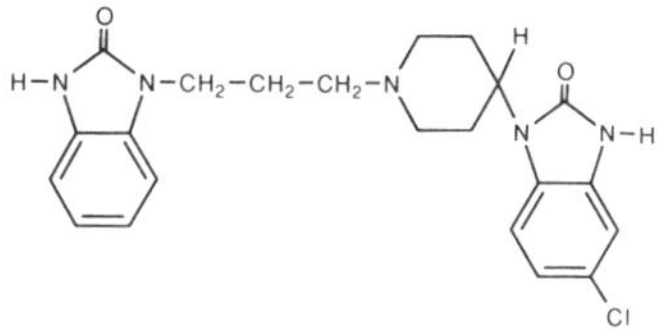

DOMPERIDONE

Domperidone is among the more complex molecules found by Janssen researchers. It is called a benzimidazole derivative due to the two benzimidazole double rings in the molecule, one at the extreme left and one at the extreme right. It is presumably the configuration of these rings that makes it difficult for domperidone to penetrate the blood-brain barrier.

A benzimidazole double ring is a joining of a benzene ring with an imidazole ring. An imidazole ring is a five-membered ring with three carbons and two nitrogens. Domperidone also has a piperidine ring, a six-sided ring with one nitrogen.

Many Janssen drugs have individual benzene, imidazole, and piperidine rings, but domperidone is one of the few Janssen drugs that combines all three rings, two of them being combined in the benzimidazole combinations.

But domperidone was expected to do more than act as an effective agent against nausea and vomiting. It has been found to improve the motility of the upper digestive system and, in particular, to restore the coordination between the stomach and the duodenum when that has been impaired. It speeds the emptying of the stomach, and acts to ease or cure the symptoms of stomach distress after meals, the so-called chronic postprandial distress.

In various clinical trials, domperidone has been shown to be helpful with such problems as belching, excessive fullness after a normal meal, frequent abdominal distension, and inability to finish a normal meal. The drug has been on the market for several years in Australia, Canada, Japan, South Africa, and Western Europe. The FDA is currently reviewing domperidone's new drug application (NDA) in the U.S.A.

In addition, there is a potentially major Janssen gastrointestinal drug presently available in several Western European countries. It is Prepulsid (cisapride) which was synthesized in 1979 by a team of chemists under Georges H.P. Van Daele. Although it is not yet approved in the United States, cisapride can sometimes be a genuine miracle drug as the story of Patrick Spinella demonstrates.

Patrick was born in 1984 with a rare condition. His intestines failed completely whenever he ate. He had to be fed around the clock because he vomited most of his food. When he was 18 months old, he was so spindly and weak that he fractured a leg when he rolled over in his crib. As a desperate measure, he was fitted with a backpack that pumped small amounts of a special nutrition formula through a plastic tube implanted in his stomach. Even then, most of this food was vomited because his gastrointestinal system could not engage in peristalsis, the wavelike contractions of the alimentary canal that carry our food through the entire digestive apparatus.

His desperate parents saw many doctors and Patrick had

surgery seven times to solve the problem. But all these efforts were unsuccessful. Finally, the parents consulted Dr. Paul Hyman, a gastroenterologist at the University of California in Los Angeles. Dr. Hyman fed Patrick two-thirds of a teaspoon of liquid cisapride. Fifteen minutes later, Patrick was given a bowl of Cheerios and whole milk, which he had never had before. He ate it all and asked for more. His parents and the doctors were brought to tears. Cisapride changed Patrick Spinella's life.

Viewed generally, dopamine in the gastrointestinal tract tends to retard the downward progress of food in the process of digestion, which may spur vomiting. A drug like domperidone tends to discourage vomiting since it encourages faster movement down the gastrointestinal tract. But the direct encouragement and regulation of downward mobility is largely the task of another neurotransmitter, acetylcholine.

Acetylcholine works by encouraging peristalsis through a sort of digestive computer, the plexus myentericus, whose neurons are everywhere in the gastrointestinal system. The nature of cisapride can be understood most easily if we look at its structural formula along with the structural formulas of haloperidol and metoclopramide.

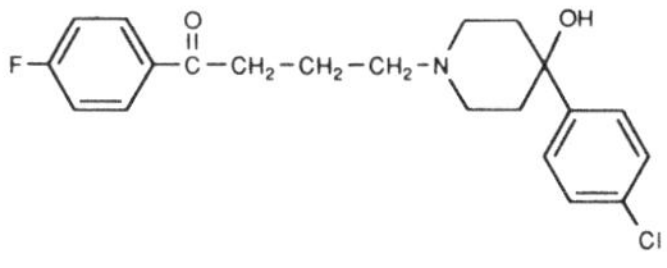

F, O, C, CH_2, CH_2, CH_2, N, OH, Cl

HALOPERIDOL

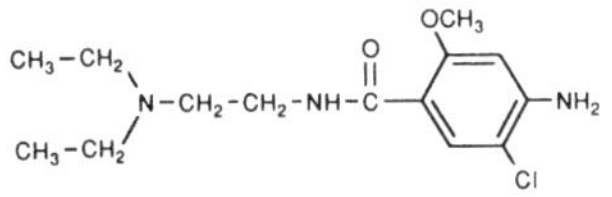

CH_3, CH_2, N, CH_2, CH_2, NH, C, O, OCH_3, NH_2, Cl

METOCLOPRAMIDE

F, O, CH_2, CH_2, CH_2, N, OCH_3, NH, C, O, OCH_3, NH_2, Cl, $.H_2O$

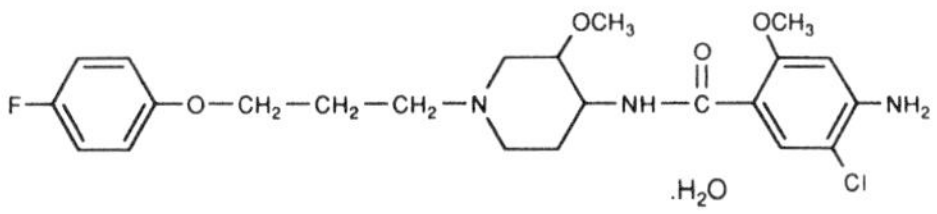

CISAPRIDE

Cisapride can be thought of as a combination of large

parts of metoclopramide and haloperidol. The extreme right-hand portion of the cisapride molecule is the right-hand side of metoclopramide while the left-hand side of cisapride is, for the most part, the left-hand side of haloperidol. But cisapride is not a dopamine antagonist. It does not produce the typical neurological side effects of dopamine receptor blockers and its action is primarily accomplished through its effect on acetylcholine.

Cisapride operates by stimulating the release of acetylcholine from the myenteric plexus to the muscle layers of the intestine or gut. This plexus is a network of small neurons which are located in the wall of the gastrointestinal tract that regulate and coordinate the complex motor events within that tract. The neurons inform each other of the events taking place at adjacent as well as remote points in the tract, and when they operate properly, the digestive process works in a very coordinated fashion.

Timing and spacing of events are programmed by the myenteric plexus. Difficulties arise when the program is not optimal. Cisapride has the faculty of stimulating the physiological release of the neurotransmitter acetylcholine from these myenteric neurons. Thus cisapride helps them steer the gut motility at an optimal level since interaction of acetylcholine with smooth muscle receptors results in muscle contraction. This stimulation with acetylcholine is done quite selectively at the gut motor level only, so cisapride does not affect gastric secretion or the urinary, genital, or cardiovascular systems. These effects can be unwanted, but they would result if cisapride, rather than being selective, simply stimulated acetylcholine release anywhere in the gastrointestinal tract.

But instead, cisapride stimulates acetylcholine release and motility specifically in the lower esophagus, stomach, small intestine, and colon. It tends to be useful in esophageal reflux disorders, in various stomach disorders, and in the treatment of clinical conditions that result from deficient motor coordination in the gastrointestinal tract. Cisapride does many of the things domperidone does and many other functions that domperidone cannot do.

The August 1988 issue of *Zoom*, a Janssen magazine, has

sketched the chemical reasoning through which cisapride was derived. Janssen researchers began by studying a compound called clebopride which was synthesized in the early 1970's and was known to be both a dopamine antagonist and to have some ability to stimulate the flow of acetylcholine. The researchers saw their task as twofold, (1) to eliminate the ability of clebopride to penetrate the brain where its unwanted dopamine antagonism could be exerted, and (2) to strengthen very substantially clebopride's small ability to stimulate the flow of acetylcholine.

A compound's ability to penetrate the brain may be ended or diminished by changing it from a lipophilic compound to a hydrophilic compound. In the case of clebopride, it was determined that the acetylcholine-stimulating or motility-stimulating part of the molecule was the right-hand part centered around the benzene ring and its substituents. Thus it was decided to make the right-hand portion of the clebopride molecule hydrophilic by attaching an OCH_3 group to the piperidine ring which marked the left-hand terminus of the portion of the clebopride molecule used for the formation of cisapride.

For the left-hand side of the cisapride molecule, various "tails" were tried and the tail which is the left-hand side of the haloperidol molecule turned out to be the most satisfactory. But the actual problem of synthesizing the molecule which is now cisapride was more complicated than is implied by saying that cisapride is essentially a combination of the right-hand side of metoclopramide and the left-hand side of haloperidol.

Two major differences between domperidone and cisapride deserve special attention. Unlike domperidone, cisapride corrects abnormalities of intestinal peristalsis. As a result, it may be useful to patients who suffer chronic constipation and pseudo-obstruction, that is, the lack of progression of intestinal contents despite the fact that the bowel is open. Another hallmark of cisapride is its ability to limit reflux from the stomach back into the esophagus. In fact, cisapride is very effective in healing esophagitis, an inflammation of the esophagus that is a severe consequence of chronic reflux.

The same property has important implications for pediatric patients. Gastroesophageal reflux not only directly causes pain and discomfort, but may also be responsible for serious respiratory disorders in children. This phenomenon explains the observation that children with chronic bronchopulmonary disease benefit from cisapride.

If preliminary clinical trials are correct, cisapride, which is already registered in Canada, Colombia, France, Great Britain, Luxembourg, Sweden, and Switzerland, may have a unique and unexpectedly useful effect on patients who suffer from cystic fibrosis. CF patients often have difficulty with their gastrointestinal tracts because the normal mucus tends to become sticky and obstruct the flow of digested products. These patients frequently experience heartburn because of the reflux into the esophagus where the stomach acid produces a very sharp burning sensation. They also have other stomach and lower intestinal difficulties, including steatorrhea or poor digestion of fats.

Cisapride's effect in cystic fibrosis patients was discovered by a Dutch pediatrician in The Hague, who had asked for quantities of cisapride for what is called compassionate use of the drug — use in patients with no alternative remedy and for whom the drug may be allowed even though it is not yet formally approved. The physician treated his patients for serious gastrointestinal problems and observed that not only were the symptoms relieved, but that typical CF disorders — steatorrhea, respiratory symptoms, and failure to thrive — improved as well. Similar observations were reported by other investigators.

Dr. Reyntjens and his collaborators have great hopes for cisapride. But, as with all drugs, the final verdict will not be in until cisapride improves the lives of many patients. That is the most consequential test for every pharmaceutical discovery. Its benefits to patients dictate its success.

Chapter 11

DON'T SURRENDER TO ALLERGIES

On any given day allergies affect tens, perhaps hundreds, of millions of people around the world. They cause symptoms and discomfort that range from the occasional cough or sneeze, or minor red spots on the skin, to a life-threatening attack of asthma or death caused by anaphylactic shock, the most severe reaction a sensitized person can suffer.

Allergies are malfunctions of the body's immune system, which works continuously to protect us against the entry of germs, viruses, and other hostile organisms and to cure us if we fall victim to one of these enemy invaders. In an allergic person, the immune system has become hypersensitive to some substance in the environment. These substances set off allergic symptoms which cause varying degrees of discomfort.

Given the discomfort and even danger that allergies cause, it is understandable that medicine has long sought drugs which would end or at least ease the symptoms. Much progress has been made, particularly against histamine, a compound produced naturally in the body which often plays a major role in setting off the symptoms of allergies. The development of the first antihistamines in the 1940's provided effective drugs which could often prevent or at least palliate allergic attacks. The histamine receptors in human tissue which potentiate allergic reactions are usually referred to as H_1 receptors, to distinguish them from H_2 receptors which are involved in the gastric secretions.

Many drugs were developed as a result of histamine research. Some of them turned out to have more important uses for the treatment of psychoses and severe depression. Others turned out to be important cardiovascular drugs. Development of antihistamines and other antiallergy drugs continues as chemists search for more effective drugs that do not cause the side effects inherent in the original generation of antihistamines. One of the most common and serious of these side effects is drowsiness which can incapacitate a person. With its usual ingenuity, the pharmaceutical industry has turned the harmful side effects of traditional antihistamines into a new class of drugs. Many of the over-the-counter sleeping pills now widely available are antihistamines, and the drowsiness they produce is a blessing to the person who suffers from insomnia. However, drowsiness is generally an unwelcome side effect to the allergy sufferer.

Dr. Paul Janssen's research in the field of allergy and antihistamine drugs began in the very first years of his independent research work and has continued up to the present. In 1955, Dr. Janssen produced Stugeron (cinnarizine), R 516; in 1967, Sibelium (flunarizine), R 14950. Eight years later he discovered Tinset (oxatomide), R 35443, and in 1977, Hismanal (astemizole), R 43512 was developed.

Over a period of approximately three decades, Janssen Pharmaceutica has produced seven antiallergic drugs, four of which are in widespread use in many parts of the world. Three drugs are still in development, being rigorously tested for their safety and effectiveness to meet the standards of the FDA and similar regulatory agencies in other countries.

How were these drugs discovered? We obtain a clue if we look at one of the earliest antihistamine drugs, diphenhydramine, better known in the United States as Benadryl. The structure of cinnarizine looks very much like an extension of diphenhydramine. Cinnarizine has essentially added a piperazine ring, an additional benzene ring, and a somewhat different group of carbon and hydrogen atoms to the diphenhydramine molecule.

Flunarizine is simply the cinnarizine molecule with two added fluorine atoms, each attached to one of the benzene

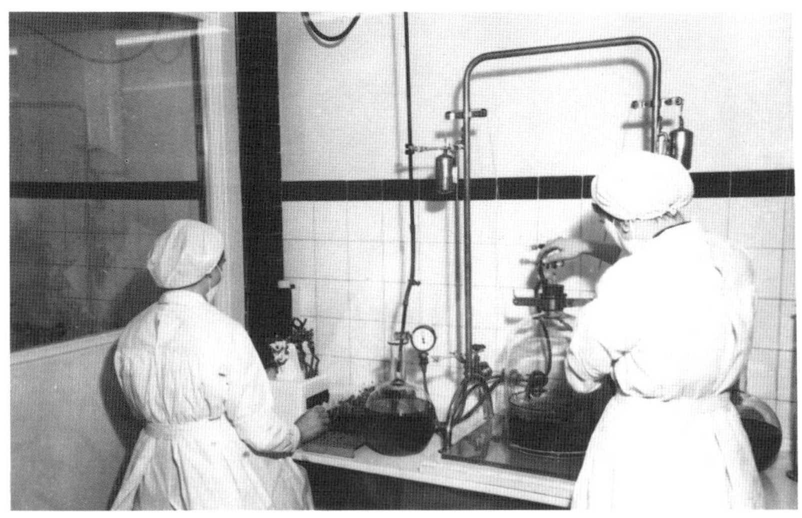

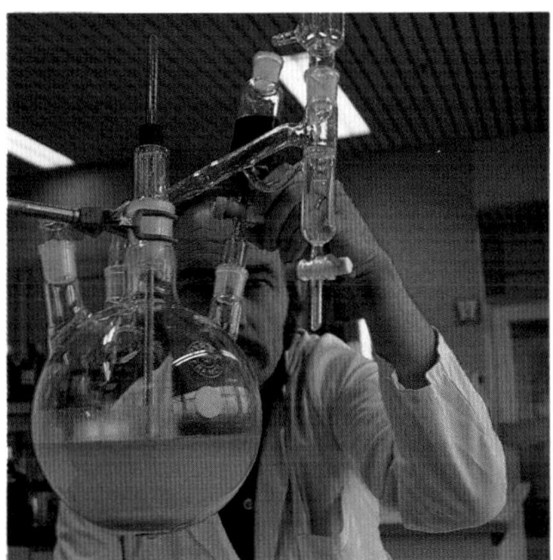

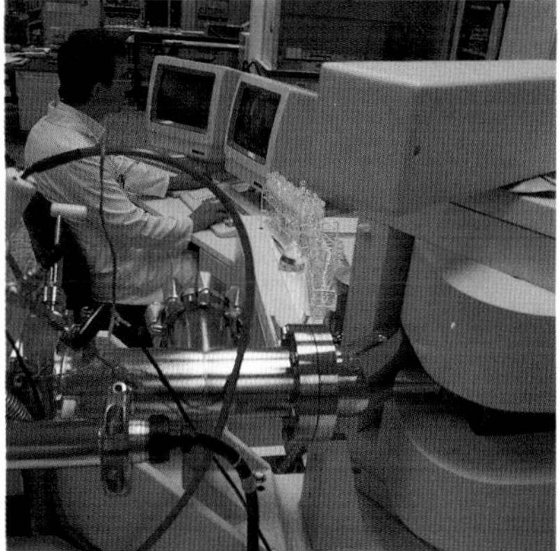

Antihistamines were first developed in the 1940's. In the last thirty years, Janssen research has grown in sophistication and has yielded seven valuable antihistamines. Among them is the new non-sedating, once-a-day medicine called Hismanal.

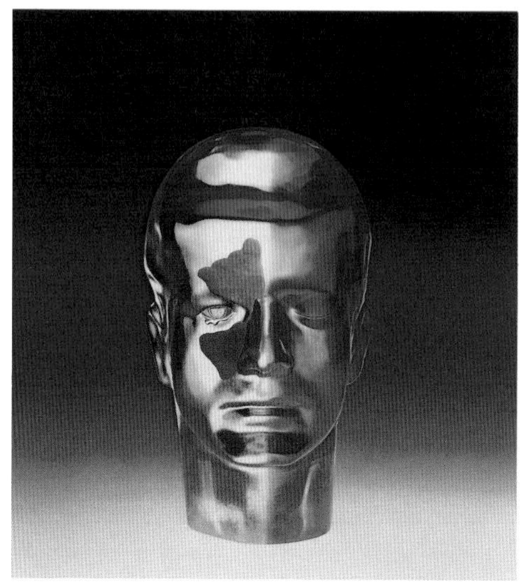

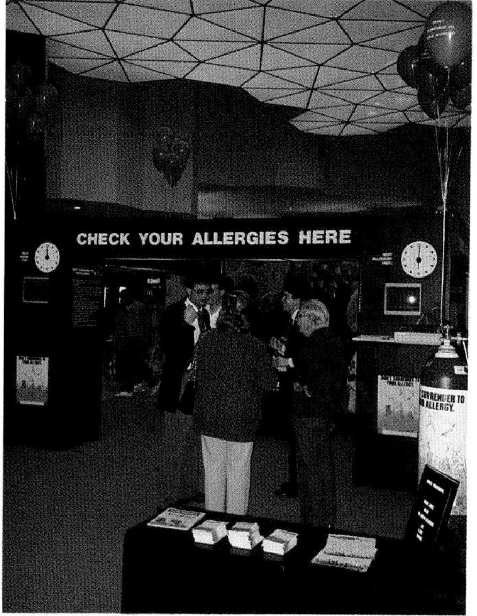

Allergies, a universal problem, range from an occasional sneeze to life-threatening asthma attacks. To communicate allergy information, an innovative program at shopping centers allows individuals to meet with an allergist, to be checked for allergies and be referred to local doctors.

rings taken over from diphenhydramine. Fluorine atoms are frequently added to a compound in order to retard the metabolism of the compound by the enzymes and other chemicals in the body fluids. Put simply, such use of fluorine is frequently motivated by a desire to make a drug effective for a longer time.

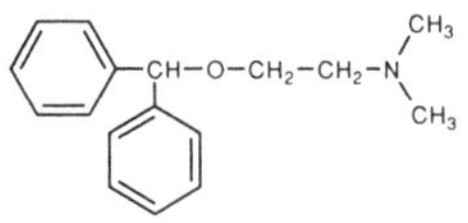

DIPHENHYDRAMINE	CINNARIZINE
FLUNARIZINE	OXATOMIDE

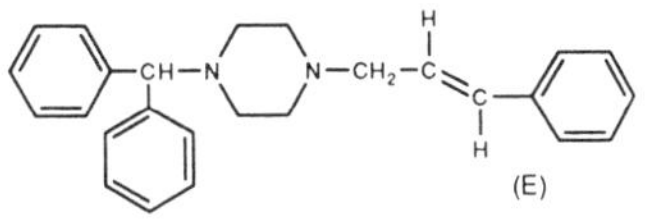

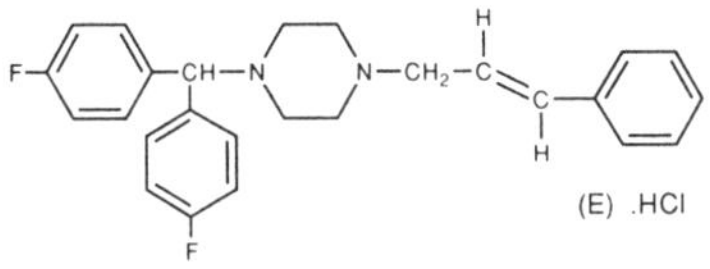

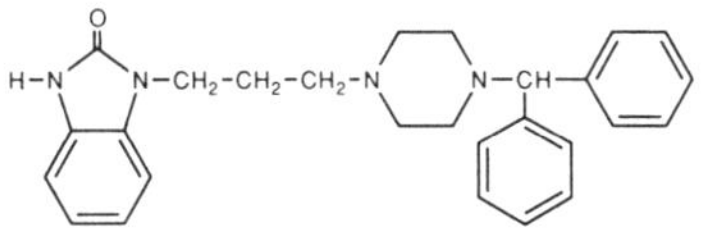

Finally, oxatomide is formed by taking the left-hand side of cinnarizine, consisting of the two benzene rings and the piperazine ring, and adding to that a benzimidazole ring instead of the benzene ring in cinnarizine. There are some changes in the pattern of carbons and hydrogens connecting the left-hand and the right-hand sides of the two molecules, and an oxygen has been inserted into the oxatomide formula.

One may be struck with the obvious similarities in the chemical structures of cinnarizine, flunarizine, and oxatomide and think that their synthesis was easy, especially after cinnarizine was found. But such thinking fails to take into account the vast number of analogue and derivative compounds that can be made starting with a particular compound.

Each of these new compounds is different; even the addition or deletion of a single atom can make a significant difference. It is only in retrospect, when we know the successful variations, that the process looks simple. To the chemists and pharmacologists who worked on these problems during the 20-year period between the discovery of cinnarizine and that of oxatomide, their labor did not seem simple nor were the resulting compounds obvious from the beginning.

No doubt when Paul Janssen planned the chemical maneuver which resulted in cinnarizine in 1955, his hope was to find a better antihistamine. Although cinnarizine and its closely related compound flunarizine have helped many patients, they have not been viewed primarily as antihistamines. Ironically, 14 years later, fate would play a trick on Dr. Janssen. In 1969 a Janssen researcher published a paper on the possible uses of this compound because of its calcium control properties. As pharmacologists and physicians worked with these drugs, cinnarizine and flunarizine were found to be very effective calcium channel blockers, affecting the movement of calcium ions in and out of the cells. Calcium channel blockers have now become an important new category of cardiovascular drugs.

Cinnarizine works powerfully to widen human blood vessels and to counteract vasoconstrictive forces. It acts primarily at the level of cell membranes — where calcium transport is very important as a control mechanism — and hence on the tone of vascular smooth muscle cells. It is widely used for prophylactic and maintenance therapy for symptoms of cerebral blood vessel spasms and arteriosclerosis. It acts against dizziness, ear buzzing, unsociability and irritability, fatigue, sleep rhythm disorders, certain types of depression, loss of memory, incontinence, and certain other disorders common in the elderly population.

Cinnarizine also helps prevent signs of vascular spasms and arteriosclerosis in the body's peripheral circulation, including such concrete ailments as intermittent blockage of the peripheral circulation, night cramps, and cold extremities. It is also helpful in preventing symptoms of disturbance of the vestibular system which controls our equilibrium and ability to remain erect. These symptoms include dizziness, nausea, vomiting, and motion sickness.

Flunarizine is used for many of these same purposes.

Additionally, it is effective in the reduction of frequency of migraine headaches. There are also some signs that flunarizine may improve the ability of a patient suffering from cerebrovascular diseases to think logically. As a result, flunarizine is used widely to improve mental functioning in the elderly.

Meanwhile, work on the new Janssen antihistamines continued, and in 1975 chemists successfully synthesized oxatomide. It combined both antiallergic — particularly antihistamine — activity and antispasmodic activity. Oxatomide is a potent antagonist of the substances that cause constriction of the bronchi which makes breathing difficult and threatens asphyxiation in a severe asthma attack.

Double-blind studies have shown that oxatomide is effective in children with chronic or exercise-induced asthma, as well as in a proportion of adult chronic asthmatics. Oxatomide is a full spectrum antiallergic agent effective against many of the substances produced in the mast cells such as histamine, serotonin, and leukotrienes. Thus, it can prevent many types of allergic reactions in addition to asthma.

The synthesis of Hismanal (astemizole) in 1977, twenty-two years after the discovery of cinnarizine, was one of Dr. Janssen's long-held ambitions. He had always wanted to find a drug which was virtually devoid of the sleep-producing property that plagued so many patients who took the earlier antihistamines. It was actually discovered unexpectedly as a byproduct of research seeking to find better antipsychotic or neuroleptic drugs.

The discovery of astemizole was most unusual. Janssen chemists were working with a group of compounds called diphenylbutylpiperidine derivatives which were originally investigated because it seemed possible they might have neuroleptic properties. Additionally this group of compounds was also found to have moderate antihistamine activity. One of them, R 39848, turned out to be particularly potent. Since R 39848 had at its core a piperidine ring joined to a benzimidazole ring by an NH combination, the chemists synthesized about 500 related compounds. Astemizole, R 43512, emerged after these 500 compounds had been tested against each other.

How were so many of these compounds screened so quickly for antiallergic properties? This technical problem was solved by a group of Janssen pharmacologists under the leadership of Carlos Niemegeers. It had been known that if a very irritating chemical mixture called Compound 48/80 is injected into a rat at a dose of half a milligram of the compound per kilogram of animal weight, this quickly causes certain body cells — the mast cells — to produce a series of harmful compounds, mainly histamine. The injection quickly produces behavioral changes in the rats and they die within 20 to 40 minutes after the injection.

Dr. Niemegeers and his associates discovered that when an antihistamine is given to a rat, the antihistamine protects the rat against death. The level of protection depends upon the particular antihistamine and the dose administered. At a sufficiently high dose, none of the rats who were given Compound 48/80 died. This test gives a means of comparing different antihistamines quickly and a way of finding the most potent antihistamine, the one that gives the most protection with the lowest dose.

Compared to a group of reference compounds, oral astemizole turned out to be the most potent protective compound tested at the time. Half the rats were saved when given astemizole at a dose of only 0.11 mg per kg of animal weight. In the testing process, it was also found that astemizole had virtually none of the sleep-inducing power associated with earlier antihistamine drugs.

Astemizole was chosen to go into clinical trials because laboratory testing indicated a superior compound. It showed potency in the Compound 48/80 test; it was effective as an oral drug; and its activity was long-acting. These tests suggested that astemizole would have a long-lasting protective effect against histamine in the human body. They are important factors in the development of a compound as an anti-allergy medication.

In the countries where astemizole has been approved, it has helped the lives of countless allergy sufferers. Most recently, in late 1988 Hismanal was approved in the United

States. The long delay by the FDA in approving Hismanal was particularly strange because in other industrial countries it is not only available as a prescription drug, but is also available in some countries as an over-the-counter drug.

Hismanal offers 24-hour protection with the convenience of one tablet, once-a-day dosing. For allergy sufferers who look to prescription medications for seasonal allergy relief, once-a-day is a simple regimen with which to comply. This means allergy sufferers can receive effective relief in the last week of their allergy season just as they did in the first week.

According to allergist Robert Lanier, M.D., moderator of the syndicated television program 60 Second Housecall, "Allergy symptoms from hay fever frequently caused by pollen from ragweed, grasses and trees plague many adult Americans. And treatment difficulties often arise from the sedating effects of conventional antihistamines."

Hismanal has been shown in clinical studies to provide unsurpassed efficacy with no sedative effect greater than placebo. Side effects have been generally mild and infrequent over the six years representing 20-million patient months of usage. Hismanal is available in 105 countries worldwide.

Looking at the structural formulas for Hismanal (astemizole) and the three antiallergy drugs still in development, levocabastine, barmastine, and noberastine, it is obvious that these four molecules have nothing in common with cinnarizine or with oxatomide. They are all independent chemical creations with very different roots that distinguish them sharply from the earlier antihistamine compounds.

Levocabastine, R 50547, is an antiallergic with H_1 antagonist activity so powerful that it may be one of the most potent antihistamines ever found. Barmastine, R 57959, which was synthesized in 1983, is both powerful and non-sedating. Most recently, Janssen chemists have synthesized noberastine, R 72075, which has a fast onset of action, is non-sedating, and needs to be taken only once a day.

Barmastine, R 57959, was synthesized as the result of a large-scale program to produce a better drug than astemizole by synthesizing a large number of astemizole derivatives. As the structural formulas indicate, barmastine and astemizole have almost exactly the same right-hand side. The one difference is that the benzene ring at the lower right of astemizole is turned into a pyridine ring in barmastine. A pyridine ring is a benzene ring in which one nitrogen atom has replaced a carbon atom. Even more astonishing, the left half of barmastine is the same as that of the left half of risperidone, R 64766, a compound that may turn out to be the best antipsychotic drug available.

Noberastine, R 72075, was derived in a completely different fashion. It emerged from a study of the complex biotransformation and metabolism of astemizole in man. One of these metabolites, the nor-metabolite, was found to be a very fast-acting antiallergic drug, but to have less potency than astemizole. Since barmastine had been shown to be more potent than astemizole, the researchers decided to study the nor-metabolite of barmastine.

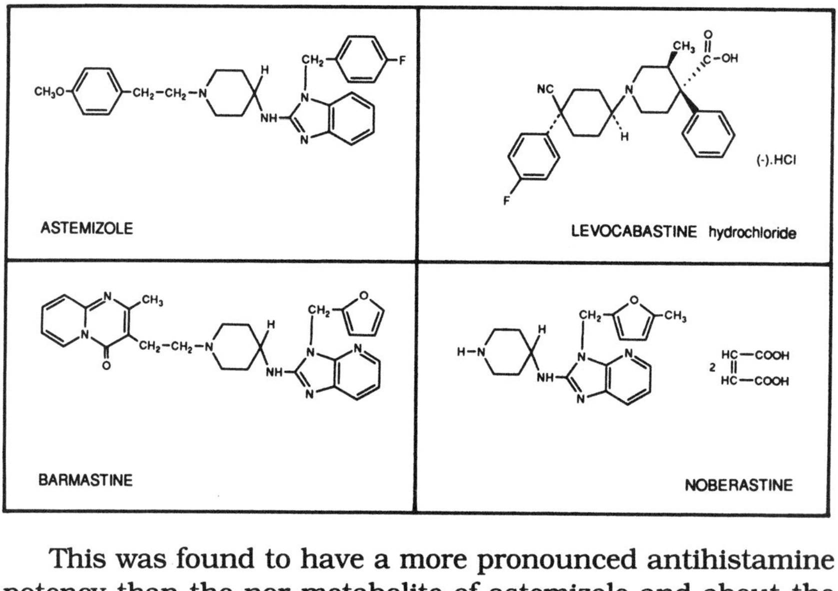

ASTEMIZOLE

LEVOCABASTINE hydrochloride

BARMASTINE

NOBERASTINE

This was found to have a more pronounced antihistamine potency than the nor-metabolite of astemizole and about the same overall high antiallergic effect of barmastine. Further manipulation of this metabolite resulted in the addition of a methyl substituent (CH_3) to the furan ring — the five-membered ring on the upper right with a single oxygen atom.

As the structural formula shows, the body of R 72075 is

essentially the right half of barmastine with the addition of a single hydrogen atom at the extreme left and a methyl group at the extreme right. And, as pointed out earlier, the right half of barmastine is almost identical with the right half of astemizole.

The resultant compound is a non-sedating, antiallergic drug with a rapid onset of action. Noberastine's duration of action is long enough so that the drug needs to be taken only once a day. It also has a large safety margin, allowing dose increases in accordance with the severity of the allergic reaction. Some Janssen researchers believe R 72075 is as close to an ideal allergy drug as can be achieved.

Since Hismanal was synthesized in 1977, the Janssen chemists had the kernel of an ideal antiallergic more than a decade ago, but it required half a decade for them to realize that. The intricate chemistry of these compounds can blind even the best chemists and pharmacologists, at least for some years. For the Janssen family of drugs, Hismanal ushers in a new generation of antihistamines. Meanwhile, for the Janssen family of researchers, noberastine is a vital compound in the development of future antiallergy products.

Chapter 12

THE CRUSADE FOR ANIMAL AND PLANT HEALTH

Dr. Paul Janssen and his collaborators have not restricted their research solely to new and better medicines to cure or at least palliate human diseases. Their research has also resulted in the development of numerous products which are useful in protecting animal and plant health.

While the usefulness of drugs is less apparent in plant than in animal protection, it is no less important. Antibiotics and antifungal drugs developed against human diseases may be useful against bacterial and fungal plant diseases as well. Janssen, however, has never synthesized new antibiotics or insecticides, so its activity in the plant protection field is limited to antifungal drugs. Furthermore, Janssen compounds used in the animal health and plant protection fields are either the same compounds used in human illnesses or are derived from the same sources from which the human drugs were found.

From the point of view of veterinary medicine there are two categories of animals: pets and livestock. Some pets are so dearly loved by their owners that they are willing to pay for high-class, high-tech, modern health care. Often, an owner desires the best, rather than the cheapest, medical care. These animals, for the most part, receive prescription drugs for their ailments through veterinarians.

But the great majority of pharmaceuticals used in animals are over-the-counter products rather than prescription drugs. Livestock management involves the breeding, care, and raising of different animals primarily for food: milk from cows, eggs from chickens, meat from cattle, sheep, pigs, poultry, and rabbits. Horses, and in some areas camels, are raised for transportation or racing. Pigeon raising is inextricably linked to pigeon racing as a hobby in many countries. Many materials for clothing are obtained from animals: wool from sheep, leather from cattle and other domesticated animals, and furs from a large variety of animals, some of them raised in confinement as in the case of mink. The progress of aqua-culture has reached the point where some fish and shellfish, for example salmon and shrimp, are now raised for market on fish farms.

Livestock raised for commercial purposes are not expected to live out their natural lives. On the contrary, the owner expects to raise these animals only to the economically advantageous point where the receipts from the sale of these animals and their products are maximally greater than the costs of further rearing. From the livestock raiser's point of view, the most attractive form of medicine is preventive medicine, such as antibiotics, antifungals, anticoccidials, and anthelmintic drugs mixed with livestock feed. These drugs are sold over-the-counter in large quantities to farmers and permit his livestock to prosper at a minimum cost until they are slaughtered.

The costs of medical care for individual animals being raised for food are unattractive to the owner. His concern with the illness of one or a few of his animals arises mainly from the worry that these few sick animals may be the first cases of an epidemic which might decimate his herds or flocks. Alternatively, such illness might lower the average production of milk or eggs or the average quality of the wool or leather being harvested.

Prescription medicines for the benefit of a sick animal are rarely wanted by owners of most commercial livestock. They make up only about ten percent of the animal health pharmaceutical business. A prize bull or a champion race horse, however, is a valuable asset and receives the best possible care, including prescription drugs.

Because of the industrialization of most livestock raising in the United States and other advanced countries, preventive medicine has become of great importance to livestock raisers, especially in the last two decades. Today's mass production chicken farms operate with 10,000 to 30,000 chickens in a single large structure. Chickens are kept in small pens where they are fed scientifically so that they can gain weight as quickly and as cheaply as possible. Then they are slaughtered for the market.

Many dairy farms have large stables in which cows are penned up and fed to maximize their milk production. Meat cattle are similarly penned and cared for so that they will put on weight as economically as possible. The crowding of animals into confined areas increases their vulnerability to disease. It also increases the threat of epidemics once disease strikes.

The Janssen interest in animal health care was a predictable consequence of the addition of veterinarians to the staff in the early 1960's when Dr. Robert Marsboom, Dr. Denis Thienpont, and others arrived from the former Belgian Congo. The first medicine to specifically address the needs of livestock care was released in 1962 as neurolept-analgesia for use during surgery in dogs and other small animals. Its constituents were a neuroleptic, fluanisone R 2028, and fentanyl, R 4263, the anesthetic. This preparation is a small-volume prescription drug, rather than a mass-volume preventive medicine.

Since 1962, animal medical work at Janssen has proliferated. At the end of 1986, of 93 original new chemical entities, 37 were already being developed or used for animal medical products. Currently, Janssen animal medicine products are available in 86 countries. In the veterinary sector of animal health, anthelmintics, drugs aimed at curing or preventing worm infections, account for about 75 percent of the Janssen animal medicine.

Levamisole, R 12564, along with mebendazole, R17635, and flubendazole, R 17889, have proven to be important and effective anthelmintics for animals. In 1974, Janssen chemists synthesized closantel, R 31520. It is now widely used in countries such as Australia and South Africa where cattle and sheep are plagued by liver flukes, a variety of roundworm which, if unchecked, causes major economic loss. Some Janssen people believe that mebendazole is the best small animal dewormer available in the world, and it is used widely against worms in horses, sheep, and dogs. Flubendazole is believed to be better and even safer than mebendazole for treating pigs and poultry infected with roundworms and similar parasites.

Levamisole is often prepared in a solution and a measured amount is applied to the back of the animal. The compound is absorbed sufficiently so that it can deal with the worms inside these animals' bodies. In 1965, levamisole was a major innovation in anthelmintic treatment, the first compound in the field that was broad spectrum, water soluble, and injectable with no resistance build up. It also enhances the performance of treated animals and has immune-modulating properties. The World Health Organization in Geneva has listed levamisole as an essential drug. Emphasis at Janssen Pharmaceutica is now on economically-oriented use of worming programs through exclusive delivery systems and slow-release devices.

There is no other company in the world with such a complete battery of original anthelmintics. Presently, there is a good deal of excitement among Janssen animal health specialists about a new compound, R 72459, synthesized in 1986. In early tests this compound, which can be used orally or as an injectable drug, seems to work almost miraculously against roundworms, tapeworms, and similar parasites. One low-dose injection seems to clear an animal's body of its worms. While there is always the problem of reinfection, any serious reinfection can be ended in the same quick manner as the first infection.

Worms are not the only causes of animal diseases arising from the invasion of a foreign organism. Protozoal diseases are also major problems in animal health. They constitute an area in which Janssen Pharmaceutica has achieved significant gains in recent years. Janssen first became active in the antiprotozoan field several years ago when it introduced Spartrix (carnidazole), R 25831. Spartrix is effective against the trichomonas family of protozoa which cause a venereal disease in cattle and serious infection of the upper gastrointestinal system in pigeons.

The Janssen Animal Health Division is now focusing on coccidiosis. This is an infection caused by one-celled protozoan parasites, some varieties of which can kill the host. These parasites pose a particularly serious problem among broiler chickens, turkeys, and rabbits raised in the crowded, factory-like conditions which are now increasingly common. Coccidiosis in these animals exacts significant economic costs.

The search for an effective drug against coccidiosis began in the 1960's and several compounds were found at the end of that decade. They were not developed, however, because it turned out that the protozoan targets quickly developed resistance to those compounds. Other companies also sought safe and effective anticoccidial compounds. A series of compounds found by Pfizer chemists about 1980 were not developed because they turned out to be teratogenic to the animals and resulted in complications including birth deformities.

Janssen chemists worked to remove the toxic and teratogenic properties of anticoccidial drugs while retaining high efficacy. They found a benzene acetonitrile series from which two potent and safe compounds were selected, clazuril, R 62690, in 1982 and diclazuril, R 64433, brand name Clinacox, in 1984. Clazuril is known as a successful single-dose anticoccidial for pigeons, mainly in the same countries where Spartrix is available.

Clinacox has turned out to be virtually the ideal anticoccidial drug. It is effective against the main pathogenic coccidia in a variety of animal species, including poultry, turkeys, rabbits, sheep, cattle, and dogs. It has very little potential for inducing parasitic resistance and therefore is expected to be useful for many years. Finally, it can be used in very low doses of one part per million or the equivalent of one gram of diclazuril mixed with 1,000 kilograms of feed.

Not only is Clinacox totally effective at this low dosage, but it offers no health threat to animals, to the environment, or to the consumers of the poultry or rabbits. The speed with which Clinacox's virtues were recognized by the animal-raising industry is demonstrated by the fact that the compound, discovered in October 1984, was available in South Africa only three years later. By the early 1990's, Clinacox is expected to be available in all or most nations in Western Europe and North America.

Another major product category in the animal protection field consists of the antifungal drugs, particularly miconazole, enilconazole, and parconazole. Different antifungal drugs are suited for combating particular types of pests in particular species.

Parconazole, for example, is very potent against the *candida* fungi which often infect the gullets of chicken and other poultry. Miconazole is very potent against the fungi causing eye and ear infections in pet animals. At the end of 1987, a Janssen antifungal drug Nilfectol (enilconazole), R 23979 — long known for its effectiveness in the treatment of dermal-fungal diseases of animals — was put to a new use, helping to defend bee colonies against a fungus which causes diseases called chalkbrood and stonebrood. This fungus infects and kills bee larvae in the honeycomb, weakening the colony, reducing its honey gathering capability, and eventually killing the colony. The utility of Nilfectol in the bee-raising market was first discovered in Yugoslavia.

A third category of animal health products from Janssen Pharmaceutica may be loosely categorized as sedatives. However, in animal health the concept is broader than the usual meaning of the term sedatives. It includes, for example, carfentanil, R 33799, which is 10,000 times more potent than fentanyl and is used in veterinary medicine to anesthetize wild animals quickly so they can be examined, treated, or moved from one place to another. Azaperone, R 1929, has pronounced sedative effects on pigs and is used to prevent injury during transportation from farm to slaughterhouse.

Azaperone is a neuroleptic and is unsuitable for cattle, which are unable to stand properly if given this drug. That problem has been solved with the synthesis of tameridone, R 51163, a $serotonin_2$ antagonist used to tame cattle and wild animals without rendering them unconscious. This permits the administration of medical care to such animals as deer, elk, and mountain goats.

There are a number of other potential Janssen animal health pharmaceuticals that are in development. Metrenperone, R 50970, is a serotonin$_2$ antagonist which appears to be active against tendonitis in animals and seems to be particularly useful for horses. The improved antidiarrheal drug, loperamide N-oxide, R 58425, seems likely to be useful in the animal health field. The gastric motility drug, cisapride, R 51619, has utility in cattle and horses where, in some conditions, there is complete immobility of the intestines. Cisapride has reversed the 80-percent mortality rate in 100 percent of the cases where it has been used. Ketoconazole, the Janssen imidazole antifungal agent, is available in various forms for animal use as a constituent in dog shampoo.

A change in strategy for Janssen's Animal Health Division took place in 1987. Pitman-Moore, a subsidiary of Johnson & Johnson, was sold to International Mineral and Chemicals Company (IMC). Its new owners remain the American representative for Janssen's animal health products. Elsewhere in the world, Janssen will continue to make available their own products and the biologicals and vaccines developed by Pitman-Moore.

The IMC connection will give Janssen Animal Health Division more coverage since IMC is also likely to develop its own products. Janssen Animal Health activities, for the next few years at least, will concentrate on the European market giving special attention to the new situation in 1992 and afterward when existing trade barriers are expected to disappear within the European Community countries. At that time, there will be one European market with a single-pricing policy and perhaps a single center for approving pharmaceuticals.

Janssen Pharmaceutica became involved in the field of plant protection around the same time as its involvement in animal health began. At first, Janssen sent some of its compounds to the government-run agricultural laboratory in Gorsem. There scientists tested the efficacy of these compounds for plant protection. The outstanding compound selected was imazalil, R 23979. In 1974, Janssen terminated its contract with the laboratory and began testing its own compounds.

Dr. Jef Van Gestel of the Janssen staff had begun testing the firm's compounds for possible agricultural use in 1973, restricting himself to *in vitro* tests. A year later, a number of the Gorsem scientists were hired by Janssen to continue their study of the Janssen compounds. Finally in 1975, Dr. Van Gestel and the former Gorsem scientists opened a special laboratory at Janssen which included a greenhouse and other facilities to perform *in vitro* and *in vivo* studies to determine the activity of Janssen compounds for various agricultural purposes.

At this time, an agronomist Benedict Duytschaever joined Janssen to survey the compounds and to assess their commercial possibilities in the plant protection field. Fifteen years later, Janssen has made a significant contribution in the protection of plants including cereals, fruits, and ornamentals, as well as wood used in construction. Janssen products prevent both partial and total destruction by fungal infection. Dr. Van Gestel continues to head the basic biological research unit. The large Janssen chemistry staff synthesizes potentially useful new compounds, and Mr. Duytschaever leads the development and commercialization of the promising compounds produced by Janssen.

The Janssen contribution to plant protection has been made in several ways. First, new effective compounds were made available. These not only did a good job of fighting fungi but also replaced ecologically and environmentally less desirable products used earlier. In seed dressings used to protect wheat, barley, and other grain seeds from fungi, the older compounds were often mercury-based and were biocides which were harmful to other forms of life or created environmental problems.

Second, the new Janssen compounds came at a time when some key fungi were developing resistance to older antifungal compounds. These new Janssen compounds are permitting continued efficacious, antifungal action despite the adaptations of fungi to older compounds.

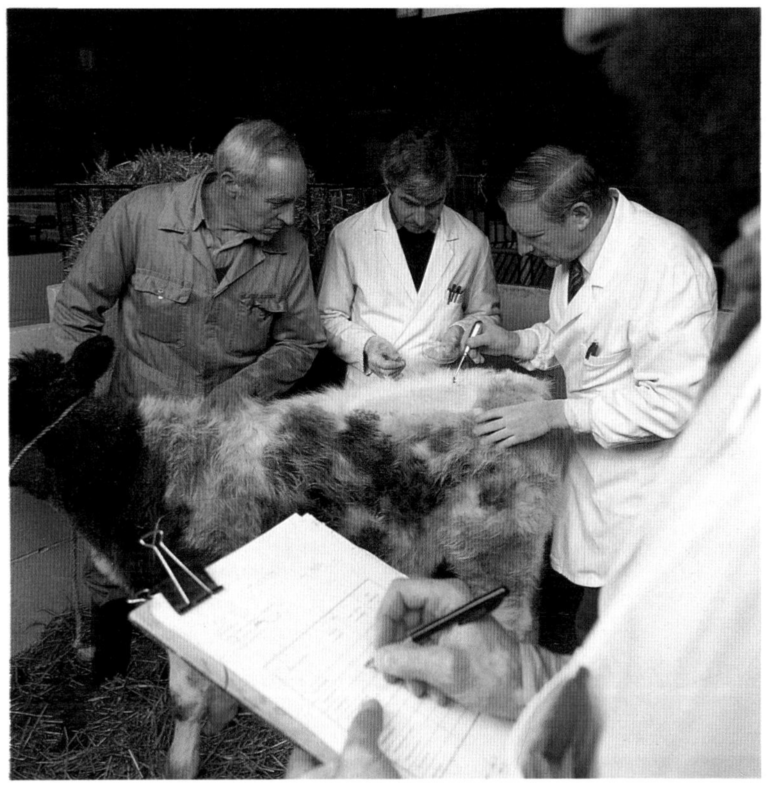

Since animal diseases can be contagious and result in severe economic loss, preventive veterinary medicine is of paramount importance in the crusade for animal health. But research involves more than treating animal diseases. It also addresses nutritional and growth studies in animal husbandry.

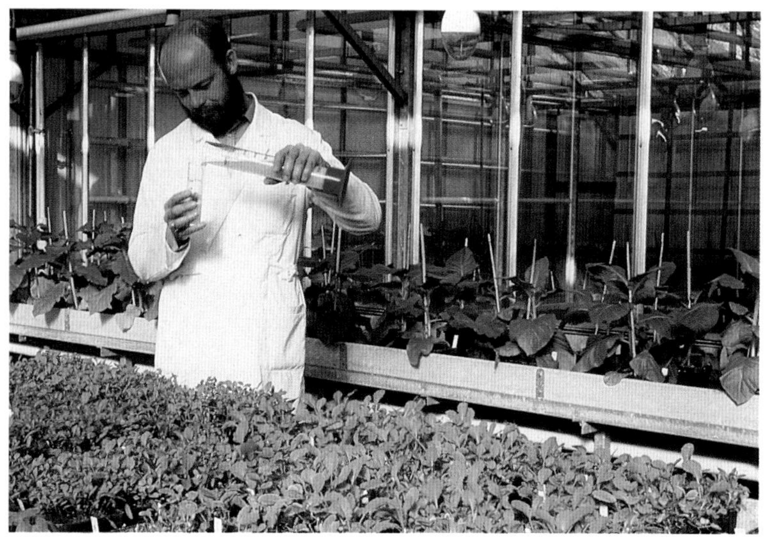

About one third of the world's food production is lost to fungi, parasites, and insects. In the last fifteen years, Janssen has contributed significantly to the protection of plants including grains, fruits, and wood. As a result, the world's food supply has increased by millions of tons.

Finally in the antifungal field, the preparations often used are combinations of compounds. In many cases, Janssen compounds are key elements in those compound mixtures. As a result, virtually all of the Janssen antifungals are distributed through other companies in the plant protection field.

The original Janssen compound employed in this area is imazalil, R 23979. It is also used in the animal health field under the generic name, enilconazole. Imazalil is an imidazole compound, similar in structure to miconazole. Imazalil is particularly active against various species of *fungi imperfecti* and *Ascomycetes* which damage many different kinds of plants. Imazalil works systemically. It can also be used in fumigation, as a fog, to control fungi in greenhouses, stables, warehouses, and other establishments which must be cleansed periodically of fungal infestation.

One of the first areas where imazalil proved its worth was in the post-harvest decay of citrus fruit. Janssen personnel were invited by Sunkist, the American citrus growers cooperative, to participate in solving fungus problems. Sunkist had found that older antifungal compounds used in fruit shipping were spoiling a significant number of the oranges, grapefruit, and lemons en route to market. This necessitated expensive and time-consuming repacking of cartons to remove the rotten fruit.

At first, many citrus companies were not interested in soliciting Janssen's help, feeling that their existing fungicides were adequate and cheaper than imazalil. But once Sunkist permitted substantial experimentation, it soon became apparent that imazalil prevented fruit spoilage and the need to repack boxes. Although this was demonstrated by the mid-1970's, it took until 1983 before imazalil was approved by the United States Environmental Protection Administration, the agency charged with evaluating the toxicological tests to determine if new compounds are environmentally safe.

Now imazalil, alone or in combination with other fungicides, is used widely around the world to safeguard many fruits during post-harvest storage and transport to market. It is employed on a large scale as a seed dressing for barley, wheat, and other grain seeds, especially in European countries with intensive agriculture and high-yielding cereal crops. One of imazalil's greatest virtues is its effectiveness at low concentration. Two grams of imazalil used in a spray can protect up to a ton of fruit. It is environmentally and toxicologically more benign than many of the compounds it has replaced. Imazalil has solved the problem of treating crops which were infected with pathogenic fungi that were resistant to older benzimidazole fungicides.

But Janssen executives were well aware that despite imazalil's excellent properties, it also had its limitations. Therefore, much effort was devoted in the 1970's to the search for effective triazole antifungals. The main objective, a usable human triazole fungicide, was found in 1980 with the synthesis of itraconazole, R 51211. But in the earlier period, three other triazole antifungal compounds useful in wood or plant protection were selected from the compounds that had been synthesized. Chronologically, these are azaconazole, R 28644, synthesized in 1973; propiconazole, R 35432, in 1975; and penconazole, R 38145, the following year. The most popular of these compounds is propiconazole.

The most damaging fungi to wood are clearly those which cause the wood to decay and ultimately to be destroyed. These include the white rot, brown rot, and soft rot fungi of many varieties. Damage is particularly prevalent where wood comes into contact with damp soil. There are also types of fungi which discolor wood without causing it to rot. These are the surface fungi which produce a superficial red, green, or black discoloration. Blue fungi produce an internal blue-black discoloration of wood without rotting it. All these types of fungi must be combated if society is to provide adequate building materials.

A Janssen publication has described the pharmacologists' search for an effective chemical weapon against wood-destroying fungi in these terms: "Day after day the potential antimycotics which arrived from the synthesis 'production line,' or had been synthesized earlier, were tested *in vitro* on the collection of fungi which attack wood. In this way hundreds of substances were distributed across thousands of culture media. Scores of them were found to have sufficient promise to take the next step: to the wood.

"The wood was then treated with the environmental substances using industrially feasible methods: spraying, brushing, immersion or vacuum-impregnation. But all on a miniature scale. Real blocks of wood were treated and then exposed to attack by all those substaining and surface fungi.

"It is not a job that you do between breakfast and lunch. A test on *Ascomycetes* and *Fungi imperfecti* takes about three weeks. A good product must keep the surface of the wood completely free of discoloration. And a test on *Basidiomycetes*, a class of fungi that rots wood, takes at least eight weeks. Untreated blocks lose about 50% of their original weight in that time. A good antimycotic can limit this weight loss to less than 3%."

Azaconazole is used primarily as a wood preservative, protecting timber and wood structures from damage and destruction by fungi. Historically, many preservatives used to be based on pentachlorophenol (PCP) or one of the sodium salts of tri-, tetra-, or pentachlorophenol. As the toxicity of these compounds became better known, the uses for many of them were restricted to improve human and environmental safety. Azaconazole has in many cases proved to be an excellent substitute for the older wood preservatives and to be far less toxic to man and his environment.

Azaconazole is also economical because it is effective in small quantities when applied in either organic solvent or water-based formulations. It also helps preserve both solid timber and wood-derived products like pressed board, particle board, and plywood. Azaconazole was first approved in Belgium in 1983. Since then, much work has been done to register azaconazole in all industrialized countries.

There are no internationally standardized environmental tests for wood preservatives. Therefore, six months or a year after a registration application has been filed, the regulatory agencies require the most diverse environmental, toxicological, and biological tests. By the beginning of 1988, azaconazole was available not only in Belgium but also in France, Netherlands, Portugal, South Africa, and Switzerland. By 1989, it is expected to be registered in Australia, Austria, Canada,

Great Britain, Italy, Japan, New Zealand, the Scandinavian countries, Spain, and the United States.

Tilt, the Ciba-Geigy fungicide incorporating Janssen's propiconazole, is used to protect cereals against plant pathogens such as powdery mildew and rust fungi. Since there are vast acreages of cereals to protect, large quantities of this fungicide are required annually. Ciba-Geigy in turn makes this fungicide available to other companies which offer it under their brand names.

Janssen research continues its ceaseless search for better antifungal drugs for agricultural uses. Experience suggests that this search will continue to be successful. Despite huge companies that dominate the agricultural chemicals and plant protection field, Janssen has made a prominent place for itself in the field. The necessities of everyday life must be protected. Janssen products will continue to safeguard the world's supply of food and wood from destruction by fungi.

Chapter 13

TOWARD A BETTER TOMORROW

At the age of 63, Dr. Paul Janssen holds the position of chairman of the Janssen Research Foundation which has laboratories and researchers in Belgium, Germany, France, England, Spain, South Africa, the United States, and to a limited extent in Japan.

Dr. Janssen was meditating over the possibility that his researchers might form an alliance with the Academy of Science in Shanghai, an institution that specializes in analyzing the chemical constitution of natural compounds. From these data, he noted, it might be possible to develop analogues that would provide new pharmaceuticals. If such a collaboration takes place this would be an entirely new field for Dr. Janssen. But his broad smile clearly indicates that he welcomes such a challenge.

Dr. Janssen's leadership is not restricted to his positions of president, director of research, and working scientist of Janssen Pharmaceutica in Beerse. He is company group chairman of Johnson & Johnson International and is called upon frequently for consultation and advice. His contributions to medicine have been formally recognized on numerous occasions by the scientific community. Awards from various universities and medical organizations around the world reflect his accomplishments.

Dr. Janssen no longer spends all of his time in Beerse overseeing the progress of his researchers and helping them when new difficulties arise. He has created an organization of scientists and business people which is able to function effectively for weeks at a time without him.

The May-August 1986 issue of *Drug Development Research* was published as a special issue commemorating Dr. Paul Janssen's 60th birthday. Subtitled, "33 Years of Drug Development Research: A Tribute to Paul Janssen," this was a festschrift, or volume of research papers written by colleagues and admirers to serve as a tribute. The journal had numerous articles about different aspects of Janssen Pharmaceutica, both basic research and development of particular compounds. Dr. Janssen's contributions to science were summarized by Staf Van Gestel and Viviane Schuermans:

"Under Dr. Paul Janssen's guidance, more than 83,000 original molecules (R-numbers) have been synthesized, which have contributed to a better understanding of the relationship between chemical structure and physiochemical properties on the one hand, and pharmacological activity and medicinal applicability on the other hand. His studies of the structure-activity relationship of the piperidine derivatives have led to the discovery of the most specific and most widely used ligands, which enabled the identification of several receptors. These discoveries have greatly contributed to the elucidation of the mechanism of action of several molecules.

"Dr. Paul Janssen's interest has been directed to critical needs of society, the diseases of the industrial world, and especially to the plagues of the Third World for which no effective cure is available. His contributions pertain to many areas of medicine: psychiatry, neurology, anesthesiology, parasitology, mycology, dermatology, allergology, gastroenterology, and cardiology. Since 1953, Dr. Paul Janssen and his team have produced over 60 new therapeutic agents available mainly in human medicine, but also in veterinary medicine and in plant protection."

In the late 1980's, there also came another tribute to Dr. Janssen and his work. The World Health Organization maintains a list of about 250 "Essential Drugs" which it regards as the absolute minimum for the health care of even the poorest country. While there is much debate about the concept of an essential drugs list, both supporters and opponents of the concept agree that the pharmaceuticals on this list are major contributions to human welfare. Five of the drugs on the list are Janssen products: haloperidol, mebendazole, levamisole, miconazole, and ketoconazole. It is a remarkable record for a pharmaceutical research organization which is only 36 years old.

Janssen Pharmaceutica looks to the future every day. The focus is on the new compounds synthesized recently and on the older compounds that have been selected for preclinical and clinical development. The Janssen research enterprise has such an abundance of promising compounds that it licenses surplus medicines to pharmaceutical houses whose research productivity is not as high. In 1989, Janssen chemists were synthesizing compounds beyond R 81000 and yet there were compounds in the R 72000 to R 74000 groups which had not been completely investigated for all potential uses.

Simultaneously, however, there were important drugs in the R 30000 and R 40000 groups which still had not been made available throughout the world. The differences among nations and among compounds in speed of market introduction depend in part upon the peculiarities of each nation's approval process and in part upon the characteristics of the drugs involved, some of which may be easier than others to develop and present for approval.

A new drug in the development phase is always a drug in danger. The nightmare that faces clinical trial specialists is the knowledge that at any time a drug may turn out to have unacceptable toxicity or to have too little therapeutic effect to continue development. So there are many drugs which in effect die during the development process. Even the drugs that enjoy a high degree of confidence by scientists are not guaranteed against unexpected developments which may prevent them from being marketed.

Data published by the FDA in 1988 show how perilous is the road drugs must traverse to gain approval. The study focused on 174 compounds whose sponsors, during the 1976-1978 period, had applied for and received the right to begin clinical trials on human beings. By December 31, 1987, only 22, or about 12 percent of these new compounds had been approved. By that date, 73 percent of these new compounds had been abandoned by the companies sponsoring them.

About 9 percent of the new compounds never actually started human trials; 20 percent were abandoned in the Phase 1 studies, 39 percent in Phase II, and 5 percent in Phase III. About 29 percent were dropped for safety reasons, 20 percent for reasons of lack of efficacy, and 24 percent because of a conclusion by the sponsors that particular compounds were unlikely to be economically worthwhile. The authors of the FDA study reported their expectation that ultimately only 35 of the 174 compounds studied would actually be approved. If this prediction is correct, only one out of five new compounds will ever become available, and four out of five new chemical entities will be abandoned.

Janssen Pharmaceutica has developed two plans to introduce new drugs in the United States. The first five-year plan from 1988-1992 calls for the introduction of Hismanal (astemizole) R 43512, a once-a-day non-sedating, antihistamine. It has already enjoyed enormous success in many countries around the world, and after more than three years of FDA consideration, it was approved in late 1988.

Second, Janssen hopes to make available domperidone, R 33812, a gastric motility drug which is a very effective drug against vomiting and other motility malfunctions of the upper gastrointestinal system. This is a compound first synthesized in 1974, yet in 1989 its approval in the United States was still some time away.

Finally, it is hoped that cisapride, R 51619, will be approved. This represents a new approach to the malfunctioning of motility along the entire gastrointestinal tract.

A second plan, spanning the five years from 1993-1997, calls for Janssen USA to introduce risperidone, R 64766; ritanserin, R 55667; seganserin, R 56413: and nebivolol, R 67555. Risperidone is the long-sought comprehensively acting antipsychotic drug which is, in the Janssen tradition, the proper successor to Haldol (haloperidol). Risperidone is effective against psychotic symptoms because it is an antagonist of both $dopamine_2$ receptors and $serotonin_2$ receptors and therefore works to eliminate both the positive symptoms of

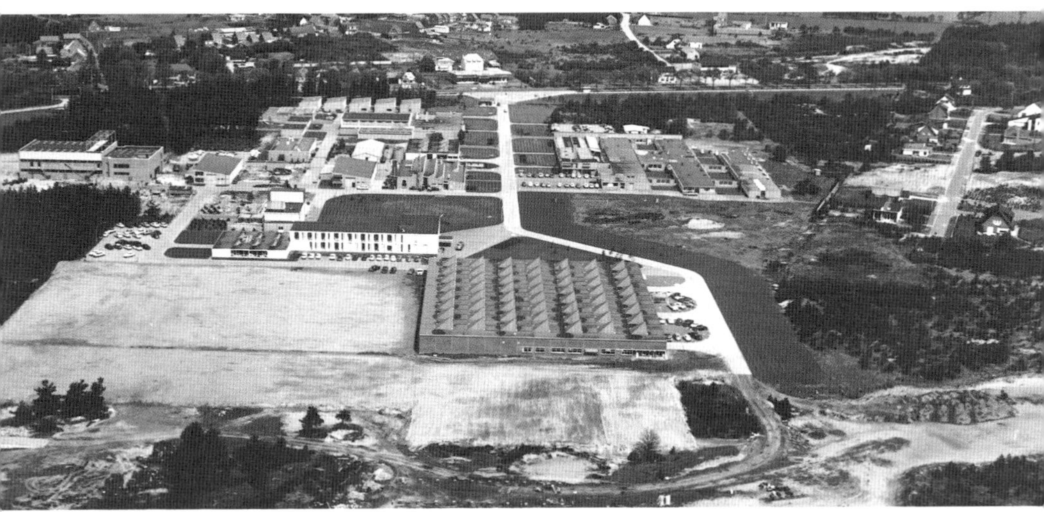

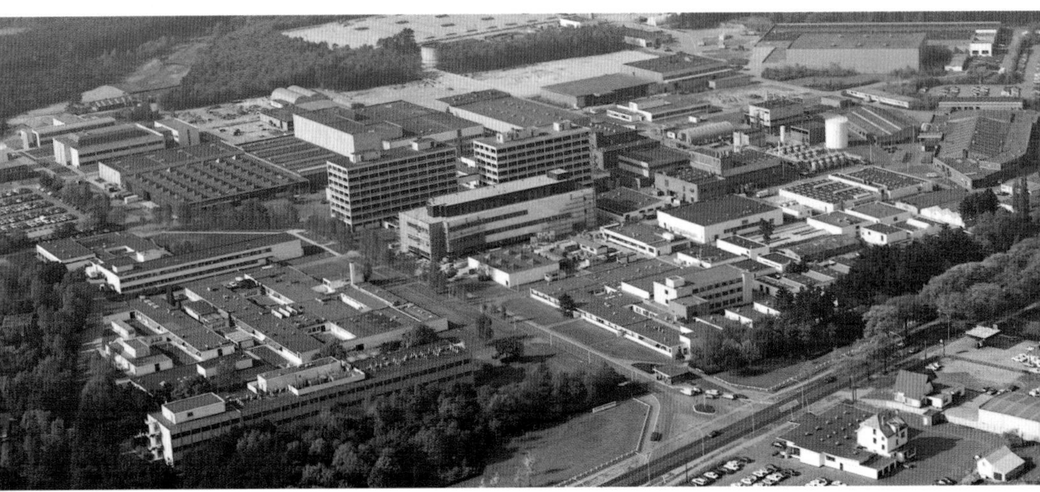

Aerial photographs of the Janssen Research Facility in 1968 (top) and in 1988 reflect the growth of the company. Each building serves a very specific function in the research process. More than 83,000 compounds have been synthesized and many new drugs now in development hold the promise of moving us toward a better tomorrow.

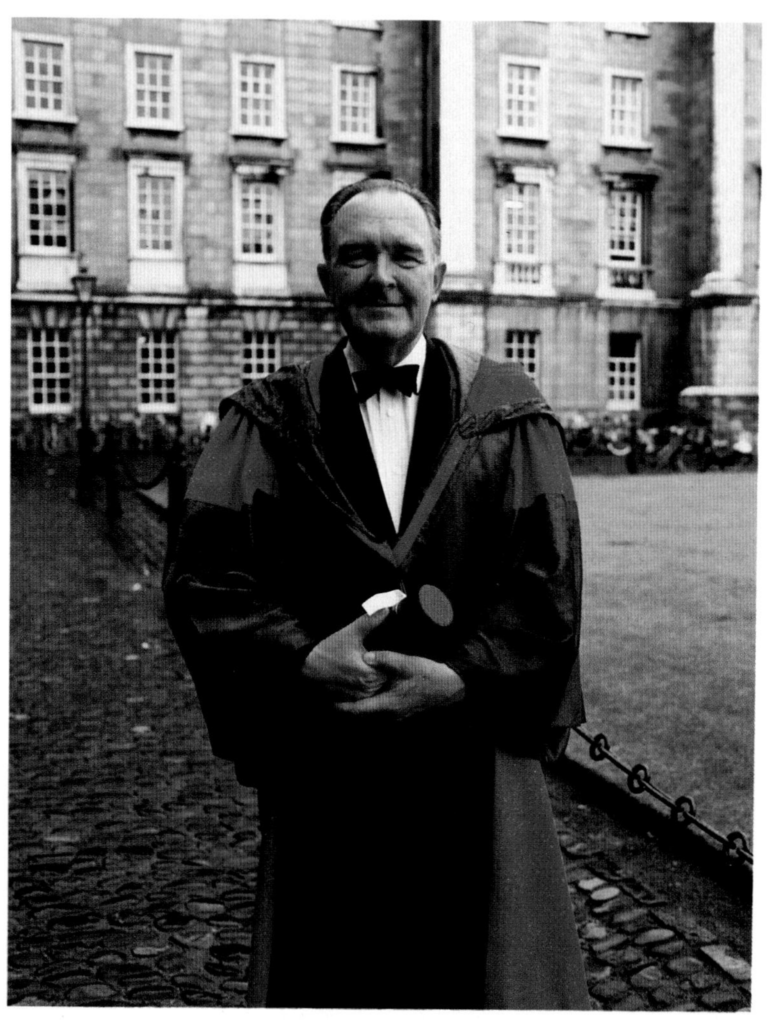

"There are still many diseases for which there is no cure and effective drugs must be found. Although we have contributed to the solutions for some of these problems, we will continue our research efforts because so much more needs to be done."
-- *Dr. Paul Janssen*

psychosis such as hallucinations and bizarre behavior, and the negative symptoms such as listlessness and failure to communicate. It seems to be almost entirely free of side effects but it remains to be seen whether that high standing will continue as clinical trials progress.

Ritanserin, R 55667, is an unusual drug that improves the quality of sleep. This action is achieved by increasing the periods of recuperative slow-wave sleep, the deep sleep that enables people to wake up feeling fully rested. Ritanserin is a $serotonin_2$ antagonist and can be used with Haldol or other dopamine antagonists to get an action against psychosis similar to that provided by risperidone in a single compound.

Seganserin is a drug similar to ritanserin. Both compounds have advantages and disadvantages relative to each other. A closer study is necessary before Janssen commits to either drug.

Nebivolol is a beta blocker but not like the several dozen beta blockers available throughout the world. Nebivolol is an extraordinarily effective antihypertensive drug. Taken alone it can normalize most cases of high blood pressure. It improves cardiac function, whereas conventional beta blockers depress cardiac function.

There are other promising Janssen-discovered drugs which may become available in the United States from Janssen Pharmaceutica, from one of the other Johnson & Johnson companies such as McNeil Pharmaceutical or Ortho Pharmaceutical, or from another pharmaceutical company through a license agreement. Janssen has a wide list of promising new chemical entities in the research and development pipeline.

Ketanserin, R 41468, is the first $serotonin_2$ antagonist to be used as a cardiac drug. It has special merit as an antihypertensive medicine for older persons. Additionally and quite independently, ketanserin also has important properties as a wound-healing agent in chronic skin ulcers.

Itraconazole, R 51211, is an oral broad-spectrum antifungal which is effective against systemic fungal infections. There is also R 66905, saperconazole, an excellent antifungal drug with better properties than those of existing medications.

Metrenperone, R 50970, a $serotonin_2$ antagonist, is useful for treating tendonitis in animals. It is also effective in helping wounds to heal.

The compound R 56865 reduces the toxicity of cardiac glycosides such as digitalis without antagonizing the beneficial effects. It also has protective effects against ischemia, inadequate circulation due to such obstructions as arterial narrowing caused by plaque deposits.

Barmastine, R 57959, is a non-sedating antiallergic compound which produces stronger action against histamine on the skin than currently available products. Noberastine, R 72075, is another non-sedating derivative of astemizole which shows both a pronounced antiallergic activity and an ideal time course of activity — its peak effect is reached rapidly but it has a short duration of action.

Sabeluzole, R 58735, is an intriguing drug. It is a cognition enhancer that increases the blood flow to organs and tissues. Impaired memory in the elderly is improved after only a single dose.

The research compound R 75251 is an androgen blocker which interrupts the normal androgen biosynthesis cascade in the body and thus apparently helps fight cancer of the prostate. The compound known as loreclezole, R 72063, is being developed as an antiepileptic and was in Phase 2 clinical trials in 1989.

The compound R 61837 is an antiviral drug which is particularly useful against the rhinoviruses that cause perhaps half of all common colds. It works by preventing the opening of the protein coat in the rhinovirus. It is that opening which allows the DNA in the rhinovirus to emerge, enter a cell, and take over that cell's reproductive machinery.

From this prototype, a series of other antiviral drugs is being developed which are more effective against most serotypes of rhinoviruses. R 77975 and compounds related to it accomplish the same preventive goal as interferon, which stimulates the body's overall resistance. However, R 77975 does not exhibit interferon's side effects.

Ridogrel, R 68070, is an orally active drug that inhibits the formation of blood clots. It is helpful in preventing reocclusion of a coronary artery or another blood vessel after a blood clot has been dissolved by a thrombolytic agent such as tissue plasminogen activator (TPA) or streptokinase.

An aromatase blocker, R 73725, may be useful against many breast cancers. Aromatase is an enzyme involved in the synthesis of estrogens, which stimulates some breast cancers. When the enzyme is blocked, estrogen synthesis is inhibited and the tumor hopefully stops growing.

Janssen Research Foundation's hunt for drugs that might be effective against AIDS began with an agreement with the Rega Institute. Its staff screened 600 molecules synthesized by Janssen in previous years for possible *in vitro* effect against HIV, the AIDS virus. These molecules were not known to be useful for any specific purpose, but they were known to be without effect in standard pharmacological assays and to cause only mild toxicity in rodents.

The prototype compound R 14458 had moderate but specific anti-HIV-1 activity. The two optical isomers of this compound were used as lead compounds from which other possibly useful compounds were sought by chemical manipulations. Finally Janssen chemists at Spring House, Pennsylvania, found R 82150 and R 82913, which turned out to be the most potent and most specific inhibitors of HIV-1 known. They have no effect on the HIV-2 virus, the cause of AIDS-2.

These TIBO derivatives turned out to have enormous power to stop the multiple cycle growth and replication of HIV-1 virus, doing so in nanomolar amounts which are 1/10,000th to 1/100,000th the amounts of these compounds needed to damage the cells being studied. By contrast AZT's margin between virus inhibition and cell damage is much lower. As reported in *Nature* February 1, 1990, R 82150 was administered to six healthy male volunteers in an amount 1,000 times the concentration required to kill 50% of the HIV-1 viruses. "The compound was well tolerated and no significant changes in haematological, biochemical or cardiovascular variables were observed." It seems likely that further research on these compounds has continued. It may be possible that the world will learn other news about R 82150 or some other Janssen compound against AIDS.

The success of Janssen Pharmaceutica testifies to the fact

that better health results from the union of brilliant researchers and the free enterprise environment. This environment has permitted Dr. Paul Janssen and his colleagues to flourish and contribute much to human welfare.

Two great dangers threaten the future of all pharmaceutical research. One is the tendency in developing countries to try to weaken or eliminate patent protection for new drugs. Yet Dr. Paul Janssen's entire career shows how central and vital patent protection is to encouraging continued fruitful research for important new drugs. Without patent protection, his small enterprise would not have become the creative giant it is today, and he would never have been able to contribute so enormously to better health.

The second threat comes from the tendency to make cost containment a priority in policy-making for the health care industry. It is true that generic drugs can often be bought more cheaply than the branded drugs of innovative companies which have financed the research. It is also true that the authorities in many countries have the power to set pharmaceutical prices at unprofitable levels even for patented compounds which may be of great value.

This kind of cost containment signals the industry that the community does not favor the tremendously expensive research needed to find important new drugs. Given that message, companies may decrease their commitment to laboratory research. The ultimate price will be paid by the sick who will not have the new drugs that intensive research could produce. The phenomenon that is the Janssen research success story could have been throttled in its cradle in the 1950's if the cost containment efforts that receive so much priority today had received that same priority 30 years ago.

Dr. Paul Janssen and the superb research institution he has created are now at the peak of their creativity and inventiveness. But it remains up to society, to the rest of us, to determine whether we really want this cornucopia of new medicines for the sick — and research institutions like Janssen Pharmaceutica — to continue functioning at the high level of productivity that has improved health care so much around the world since the 1950's.

AFTERWORD

By Jack B. McConnell, M.D.

The hallmark of scientific research today, biological as well as physical, is the increasing rate and pace of change. Events are moving so quickly that it is difficult to measure the changes they produce. Science is being transformed into technology at an ever increasing speed. In the past, science and technology operated independently, with useful scientific discovery put to practical application only after decades of development. Today the gap between science and technology, between understanding nature and using that knowledge to reorder the natural world, is becoming ever shorter.

For instance, it took 51 years between 1830 and 1881, before Michael Faraday's findings that a moving magnetic field could make an electrical current flow in a wire until the first practical electrical generator was developed. It was 40 years before Einstein's formula showing the relationship of matter and $E=mc^2$ until the first atomic bomb was detonated. That period spanned from 1905 to 1945.

There was a 20-year span from 1953 to 1973 between the discovery by James D. Watson and Francis H. Crick of the molecular structure of DNA until a practical application was found. In 1973 scientists transplanted genes from one organism to another. In 1957, Leo Isocki discovered that electrons can tunnel through solid barriers in tiny electrical devices. In 1963, six years later, this effect was first applied commercially in making semiconductor diodes. So we have four examples: the generation of electricity taking 51 years, the atomic bomb taking 40 years, genetic engineering taking 20 years, and semiconductor diodes taking six years.

Dr. Frank Press, President of the National Academy of Sciences, suggests that we are in THE GOLDEN AGE OF SCIENCE. The rate and pace of discovery will increase, and the translation of scientific discovery into technology and then into products will parallel that pace.

At a recent conference, someone suggested that more changes

will occur in our society as a result of scientific discovery over the next 20 years than have occurred over the past 200 years. Many of those discoveries will impact the health care field.

Life expectancy in the United States in 1900 was 48 for males and 52 for females, or approximately 50 years of age for the population in general. In 1986, the life expectancy had risen to 72 for the male and 78 for the female, or about 75 years for the general population. We have added 25 years or 50% to the average life expectancy in less than a century. Never before in the history of mankind has anything like that been achieved.

Today more people reach the age of 65 than were born in 1987. We are now reaching the point where we can begin to think about reaching for the maximum life span. In ancient Rome, the life expectancy was approximately 25 years of age. In contrast, the grandchildren of today's generation in the U.S. are projected to live to the age of 100. Staying healthy over that period of time and dying of old age, rather than illness, will become more commonplace.

There are several reasons for the increased longevity. One of America's favorite pop philosophers, Woody Allen, has said, "Some people try to achieve immortality through their offspring and it works, but I prefer to achieve immortality through not dying." The more serious reasons for longevity include improved sanitation, and it is a sad fact that sanitation engineers have received less credit for their contribution than they merit. The ability to provide clean, potable water and the ability to easily manage refuse has contributed immensely to our longevity. Also, improvements in nutrition, diagnosis, treatment, health care education, and health care delivery as well as our research and development system have added to our longevity.

Of all of these, the most important is our dynamic research and development system. Technology will be the driving force of the health care system for decades. It is the agent that will create significant changes in the way medicine is practiced and health care is delivered.

The best perspective on this is gained by reviewing the events of the last 40 years. In 1940 the ten leading causes of death were, in descending order, cardiovascular disease, cancer, stroke, pneumonia, accidents, tuberculosis, diabetes, suicide, syphilis, and gastritis. In 1980, just before AIDS was first observed, three of those diseases had been dropped from the top ten list: tuberculosis, syphilis, and gastritis. They were replaced by three other diseases: chronic lung disease, the result of smoking and air pollution; liver disease, the result of the excessive intake of alcohol and other chemicals; and homicide, the result of the intense and aggressive society in which we live. All three are reflections of the way we manage our lives and our environment.

In that same 40-year period, there have been two technical revolutions. The first, the pharmaceutical/chemical revolution, occurred in the 1940's and 50's. In that short span of twenty years there appeared on the health care scene penicillin, tetracycline antibiotics, diuretics, steroids, tranquilizers, and anticancer drugs. These have had an enormous impact on reducing the morbidity and mortality due to common diseases.

For instance, in 1940 every state in the U.S. had, by mandate, a tuberculosis hospital; now there are none. These sanitoria have been closed as a result of antitubercular drugs. The polio vaccine allowed us to escape the threat of the crippling polio virus. Our concern moved from more and finer iron lungs into the area of preventive medicine using the polio vaccine.

Steriods played an enormous part in the management of autoimmune diseases, particularly rheumatoid arthritis. As a result of antipsychotic drugs, we were able to release three-quarters of the patients from psychiatric institutions. With the advent of anticancer drugs we have been able to produce long-term remissions in several cancerous conditions.

Several of the dreaded childhood diseases have been brought under control. Improved therapeutic agents allowed us to control diseases such as scarlet fever, diphtheria, and whooping cough, while awaiting effective vaccines for essentially all of the common childhood diseases. Through the cooperation of the international medical community, we have managed to eliminate smallpox. The last case was reported in 1979. The scientific discussion has shifted from the discussion of smallpox as a threat to society to deciding whether to destroy all of the laboratory samples of the smallpox vaccine or save them as archival samples for future scientific initiatives.

The second revolution, the technical revolution, occurred in the 1960's and 70's and to some extent is still continuing. However, it reached it's peak during that period of time. This revolution was based on the technologies that grew out of advancements in physics and engineering. During that short 20-year period, there appeared on the health care scene lasers, ultrasound equipment, cardiac pacemakers, fiberoptics, nuclear cameras, heart-lung machines, dialysis equipment, artificial joints, automated laboratories, patient monitoring systems, computed tomography, and magnetic resonance imaging.

These have made their own impact on our health care system. Pacemakers have added years to the lives of cardiac patients. The heart-lung machine has opened the way for several different approaches to the treatment of cardiovascular disease. Dialysis equipment has extended the lives of end-stage renal patients. No one can imagine practicing medicine in hospitals without an automated laboratory or the intensive care patient monitoring systems which brought into being coronary and intensive care units.

Ultrasound, the nuclear-camera, computed tomography, and magnetic resonance imaging have transformed the field of medical diagnostics. Simple outpatient diagnostic procedures have replaced inpatient hospital procedures due to these advances. These less invasive procedures have had an impact not only on the hospital department of radiology but also on the surgical department, where elective and exploratory surgeries have been reduced significantly. As a result of the introduction of ultrasound, computer tomography, and magnetic imaging, some radiology departments are changing their names to department of imaging because many of their current technologies have less to do with X-rays than the use of different imaging systems to explore the body noninvasively.

One of the more recent results in the continuing instrumentation revolution is the emergence of the Uvar system. It uses a photoactivated material, 8-methoxy psoralen, which is administered orally to the patient. After a lapse of two hours, the patient's blood is circulated extracorporeally. The red cells are separated and returned to the body, and the white cells are routed through an ultraviolet irradiator, where they are rendered non-harmful by the UV radiation.

The third technical revolution is the biological revolution based on genetic engineering and molecular biology. The early results from this technology whet our appetites and have given us a foretaste of what to expect. For instance, tissue plasminogen activator, or TPA, dissolves the thromboses or clots that cause a myocardial infarct or heart attack. Synthetic growth hormones have been developed for use in children with growth deficiencies. Genetically engineered insulin is more biocompatible than animal-derived insulin. Erythropoietin is now being used to boost the red blood cell count allowing the patient to avoid the necessity of blood transfusions.

A plethora of technical opportunities have emerged out of molecular biology technology and have provided a stream of new options and opportunities to interact with the disease process. For example, monoclonal antibodies, proteins that act with a high degree of specificity, can be delivered to the diseased tissue for early diagnosis and treatment. Its application to cancer and cardiovascular disease, the two leading causes of death in hospitalized patients, are in the forefront of current research and development. The applications for both diagnosis and treatment are virtually limitless.

Dr. Michael DeBakey, chairman of the Department of Surgery at Baylor University Medical School, in a recent interview said, "Atherosclerosis remains the biggest unanswered question and mystery in cardiovascular disease. If we could solve that problem, we could eliminate heart disease." Recently, researchers discovered a new amino acid, aminomalonic acid, which is present in the atherosclerotic plaque in direct proportion to the severity of the disease. Ortho Pharmaceutical is developing a monoclonal antibody to the aminomalonic acid and is in the process of developing a test that, for the first time, will allow the medical profession to determine, noninvasively, the presence of atherosclerosis, its location, and the severity of the disease. It is also hopeful that a technique will be developed to remove the aminomalonic acid from the plaque, thereby destroying the plaque deposits and restoring the vessels to their full healthy states.

Monoclonal antibodies are used extensively in the diagnosis, and to some extent, the treatment of cancer. Work with animals shows that we can demonstrate not just the presence of the primary site for cancer, but also its distribution along the lymph chain or the metastasis of the cancer. The technique is so exquisite that, by using a monoclonal antibody tagged with a radioisotope, we can demonstrate the presence of metastatic cancer sites long before the pathologist can determine if slides contain cancerous tissue using traditional laboratory techniques. The monoclonal antibody technique is being used now to determine the presence of cancer, the extent of its metastasis, and whether anticancer therapy is having an impact on the disease.

To a somewhat lesser extent, monoclonal antibodies are being used in anticancer therapies. The antibody is tagged with an anticancer drug or an anticancer radioactive material. They are injected into the body and the monoclonal antibody carries the anticancer agent to the site of the cancer. A profile of monoclonal antibodies are being developed to colo-rectal cancer, cancer of the stomach, cancer of the pancreas, ovarian cancer, prostatic cancer, and certain cancers of the brain. In addition, dramatic results have been demonstrated in a few patients using monoclonal antibodies in the treatment of malignant melanoma.

One of the most exciting scientific activities is the program to map and place in proper sequence the DNA of the human genome. The human genome — a word developed from GENe and chromosOME — consists of our 23 pairs of chromosomes, 50,000 to 100,000 genes, and 3 billion pairs of DNA. The DNA data in the genome is equal to the letters of print in 13 volumes of the *Encyclopaedia Britannica.* The fully mapped and sequenced genome will be a dictionary of information of the body. It will provide us with the basic information of the form, function, condition, and diseases of mankind.

The human genome of each of us is unique, but we differ from one another by only one DNA element in 1000. This small difference (one-tenth of one percent) in the arrangement of the DNA accounts for the seemingly large differences between each of us. The difference defines the form, shape, condition and, to a large extent, the diseases of each of us. The information and data contained in the human genome will make it possible for the scientific community to develop novel approaches to the diagnosis, treatment, and prevention of essentially any disease.

The promise of the future of medicine resides to a large extent in the work of those now involved in mapping and sequencing the human genome and the expertise of those such as Paul Janssen, who will be capable of transforming the information and data into useful products for the diagnosis and treatment of disease. We live on the edge of time when no disease will be unconquerable. Cancer, arthritis, diabetes, cardiovascular disease, and even mental illness will yield their secrets and be brought under control.

As exciting as this sounds, it will not be without its costs to society. To begin with, the program to map and sequence the human genome is the largest and most costly effort ever attempted by the field of medicine and biology. It is estimated to cost $3 billion over a 10-year period.

Society has already raised its concern with the program. There is a sense that we are uncovering the very essence of humaneness. People are uneasy about the ethical issues regarding the possibility of abuse as well as their concern for the privacy of the information of a patient's genetic fingerprint. The medical and biological community must address these questions early on in order that society can become a partner in this joint effort.

The future of medicine and biology has never been more promising. We are in a position to build on the enormous contributions of such scientists as Paul Janssen. The next 20 years will see significant strides against many of the diseases that have been resistant to our best efforts. We can expect as much progress in the next two decades in the diagnosis and treatment of allergies, arthritis, cancer, diabetes, cardiovascular and congenital diseases as we saw in the recent past when we eliminated smallpox, controlled tuberculosis, learned to manage many of the mental illnesses, conquered polio, and developed new techniques and materials for eye problems and cardiovascular diseases. The biggest question is whether society is prepared for the changes, which will come at an ever increasing rate and pace of change.

Index

E

F

G

H

I

J

K

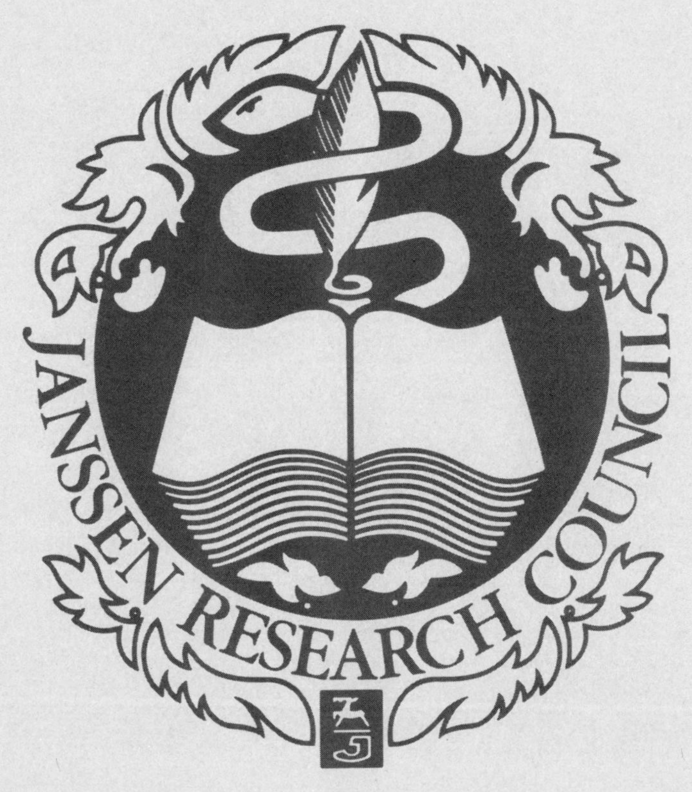
JANSSEN RESEARCH COUNCIL

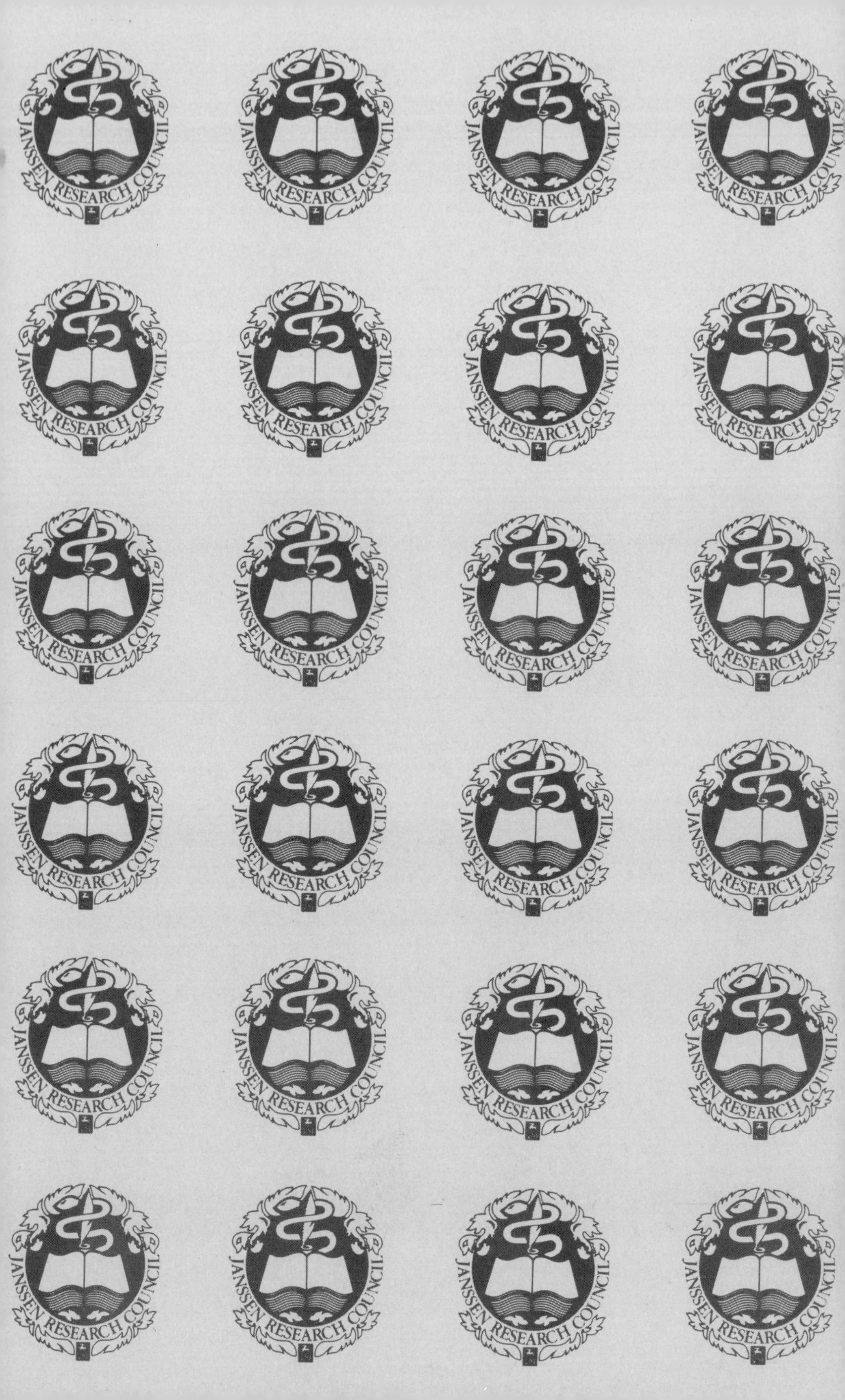
JANSSEN RESEARCH COUNCIL